MW01232580

Manipulation

The best Techniques to Influencing People with Persuasion, NLP, Dark Psychology, Analyze People and Mind Control

Daniel Peterson

Table of Contents

Introduction to Manipulation

Congratulations on purchasing your personal copy of Manipulation: The Complete Step-by-Step Guide on Persuasion, Manipulation, Mind Control, dark Psychology and NLP. Thank you for doing so. The following chapters will discuss some of the many ways you can manipulate the thoughts, beliefs, and behaviors of others and how you can recognize when that same manipulation is happening to you. You will discover how important our step-by-step guide is to identifying manipulative strategies and techniques that are being used to persuade you to do another's wished, and how quickly you can turn the tables and apply those same steps to achieve your desired outcome.

Manipulation is a topic that most people are going to turn their noses up at. They do not like the idea that comes with it, and they assume that they are above and beyond using these kinds of techniques. As we will discuss later on in this guidebook through, each of us uses manipulation in some form or another to get what we want, even though most of us are not going to do it at the expense of someone else in the process. To help us out with this we need to first take a look at manipulation and what it is all about. Manipulation is going to be the practice of using some indirect tactics to control the relationships, emotions, decisions, and even behavior over the target and how they react to things. This is often going to use a lot of different options that you are allowed to use including persuasion, mind control, deception, and more to get what they want.

Most people are going to use some form of manipulation at some point or another in their lives. For example, if you have ever had a day that wasn't going well or you weren't feeling that good, but you told someone who asked that you were doing "fine" then this is a form of manipulation. This is considered manipulation because it is going to control the perceptions and the reactions that the other person has concerning you. Even if you did it to avoid a confrontation, to avoid having someone pity you or some other reason it still changed these perceptions of you. Manipulation, at least the way that we often think about it, and the manipulation that is used in dark psychology, is going to have consequences that are often more insidious. This can sometimes include some form of emotional abuse, especially if the manipulator is in an intimate relationship with the other person. This is why a lot of us assume that all forms of manipulation are bad, but we will hold this opinion, even more, when we see that it harms the mental health, emotional health, and physical health of the other person who is the target.

While people who are the manipulators are going to do this to their target because they want to have some control over their own surroundings and environment, it is true that the urge to do the manipulation is going to stem from some anxiety and fear that is deep down. In any case, it is not going to be seen as a behavior that is all that healthy for either party. Engaging in manipulation is going to seem like a great idea to the one who is manipulating. It allows them to gain the control that they want, and they get to receive whatever they wanted in the process. However, when they use this tactic, it is not only going to cause some harm to the other person, the target, it is going to make it hard for the manipulator to connect with their own authentic self and get the benefits that come with that.

Chapter 1: Introduction to Advanced Manipulation

Now that we know a bit more about the importance of the analysis of your potential target of manipulation it is time to move to the second step of influencing other people. And this second step is going to be all about manipulation. Once you have taken a bit of time to successfully learn about your potential target, and you have been able to do a full analysis on the other person, it comes time for you to actually manipulate them. Manipulation is the part where you are going to start planting the seeds in the mind of the other person, your potential target so that you are able to get them to start agreeing with what you want them too. There are a variety of different tactics that you are able to use when it comes manipulating the target. When you are able to pick out the manipulation that includes a few different tactics, and that will allow you to gain the agreeance and acceptance of the subject that you are working with. You want to really rely on the analysis to make sure that you pick out the right technique that you want to use on your target.

Never try to work on the manipulation before you have a chance to do a good analysis. This is tempting to do for a lot of beginners. They assume that they can just jump right in and start using some of the techniques that they have learned along the way and that it will all be just fine. But this is a horrible way to get things started. If you don't do the analysis first, you will end up using the wrong kind of technique when it comes to manipulation, and you will waste time, find yourself exposed, and really lose out on the goal that you want. Even if you only have enough time to spend a few seconds or a few minutes on the analysis, like what may happen if you are in sales, you still need to take that time first. Using the wrong manipulation tactic on one of your targets, which is something that is likely to happen if you don't plan things out and think them through, is going to end badly for you and can make manipulating that target, and many others who are in your sphere of influence, really hard. If the target is able to figure out what you are trying to do, they will not be happy. Even if the manipulation is meant with no harm and would benefit both of you if the target feels that manipulation is there, then they are going to keep far away from you, and there will usually be some anger in the process. This all comes together to end with you having no chance of success with manipulating that target now or in the future. While we are spending our time in this guidebook talking about dark psychology and how to use manipulation, you have to make sure that you use that analysis above, and the persuasion that we will talk about below, in order to make it all work out well for you. Because of this, it is important to not only find the right manipulation technique to help you out, but you also need to learn more about what works for the other person and what may turn them off from talking to you in the first place. Only then will you be able to see manipulation actually benefit you.

Many people are going to have a pretty negative view when it comes to manipulation and how it is going to affect them. They assume that they have never used manipulation at all and that manipulation and the techniques that go with it have nothing to do with them at all. But think of it this way, have you ever tried to word a phrase or a request in a certain way in the hopes that the other person would help you out? Have you ever told a little white lie to get out of trouble, or to spare the feelings of the other person? If you are able to answer yes to any of these, then you have used manipulation. Most people are going to think about manipulation in the negative term, and we are going to show a few examples through this guidebook of techniques that are going to follow along with this as well. This kind of manipulation is just going to benefit the manipulator. It has no benefit for the one who is being used. They may get hurt physically, mentally, and emotionally along the way, and it doesn't really matter to the manipulator. In some cases, the manipulator wants their target to get hurt because it ensures that they are able to get more of what they want along the way.

However, the manipulation that we usually bring out on a regular basis is not going to be this bad. We often want to get something, but we will do it in a way that is going to be mutually beneficial to us and to our targets, or at least in a way that the target is going to not get hurt. When a cars salesperson tries to sell a car, they want the customer to find a good vehicle that they like. This makes the customer happy and makes the salesperson happy because they make some money. When you want someone to help you with a report, you are hoping to get some help, without any harm coming to the other person. This is the difference. It is all about intention. If the manipulator wants to get something regardless of how it is going to affect the other person, then this is seen as dark manipulation, something that is generally seen as a bad thing by most people. But if you are just hoping to get the manipulation to help you get what you want, and you don't want the other person to get harmed in the process, then this is going to be something that is not frowned upon quite as much by those around you. Manipulation is going to be something that is seen in a negative light, but you will find that there are times when we will be manipulative without really trying to cause some harm. But that doesn't mean that some form of manipulation wasn't used at some point or another. Learning when we have used manipulation and some of the different techniques that you are able to use to go along with this will make a difference in who you are able to manipulate, how you are able to manipulate them, and more.

With that said it is important for you to remember what manipulation is. We spent a bit of time talking about this in the first section of this guidebook. But remember that with this part, we are working to plant a few seeds in their minds. This is meant to ensure that the target is going to start thinking about the things that you are saying, and will start to see why it is a good idea to agree with you. Even though you used a variety of tactics to make this happen the target is going to reach this through methods that make them feel they were the ones who came up with this decision on their own.

Chapter 2: Types of Manipulation

1. Positive Manipulation.

We always think of positive reinforcement as a good thing, but malicious people can also use it to manipulate their victims. The fact is that we all use positive reinforcement in one form or another. Parents use it to get their kids to behave properly, teachers use it to make their students more interested in school, bosses use it to encourage productivity, and partners use it to modify each other's behavior in relationships. It is an integral part of our social interactions, but it only becomes a problem when it's detrimental of the person it's being used on. The answer is a thumping yes! Constructive manipulation can be used for transforming negative energy into a positive experience through physical, psychological and spiritual attributes of your personality. Imagine trying to manipulate a drug addict to give up drugs or a binge eater to start eating in a healthier fashion. Now that's not so bad, is it? You are resorting to positive or constructive manipulation to get someone to do what is good for them.

Positive or constructive manipulation has been occurring since ages. What do you think Jesus Christ, Martin Luther King or Mahatma Gandhi were doing when they drew people like magnets? They restored to spreading a highly positive energy through their own fine example and actions to lead others on the same path of equality, justice, humanity, and brotherhood. Would you call them manipulators? Not in a negative sense but they did positively influence or manipulate people through their hypnotic personalities, words, ideas, and living examples to learn important lessons of life. Think about this for a minute. There are several times in your life when you've felt compelled to reach out to someone that needs your assistance. Yet, for several reasons, he or she has turned down you straight-laced attempts for help. Is it bad then if you manipulate them to comply for their own good? Your motives can be hardly ascribed as selfish or self-fulfilling in such a scenario. The tactics you use can also be barely labeled as devious, wicked or crafty. We are all familiar with the term: "desperate times call for desperate measures." Sometimes approaching people to convince them about what is good for them in a straightforward manner falls flat. In such a scenario, when you've tried everything in the book to persuade them positively, the only communication tactics you may have to resort to may be the ones that are viewed as downright crafty or evil. The intent is precisely what distinguishes negative manipulation from constructive manipulation. In the latter, your intent isn't to twist the other person to suit your will. It is only a means to get past their stubborn, obstinate and illogical defense mechanisms. Let's take an example of how this works.

You have a childhood friend (let's call him Peter) you deeply care about. You grew up in the same neighborhood, went to the same school and your families have been thick too. You've learned through a mutual friend that Peter is about to sacked from work owing to deteriorating performance that can be traced back to him being abandoned by his partner for another man. Peter was planning an elaborate wedding ceremony with his ladylove when she ditched him a few days before the wedding and eloped with another man.

Peter felt betrayed, hurt and broken, which made into slip into a state of depression. This is now taking a toll on his professional life and affecting his performance at work. As a friend, you suggest that before anything more untoward and disastrous happens, Peter go and meet a counselor to seek some solution for his situation. Peter vehemently denies that anything at all is wrong with him and refuses to fix an appointment with a counselor. No amount of persuasion, cajoling or pleading works.

As a childhood friend, you are utterly concerned about his condition. What do you do next to bypass this obstinate approach by Peter? Overcome by absolute desperation, you speak on how a co-worker's son slipped into a coma for days before he got back to living a normal life following a near-fatal accident. You talk about how your co-worker was deeply affected, disturbed and depressed throughout the time his son was in a coma. The expressions, tone of your voice and words are carefully chosen to convey the right emotions. You then go on to state how his performance at work was an absolute disaster, and he was on the brink of losing his job.

Then you masterfully and carefully introduce how the co-worker agreed to meet a therapist on your suggestion, which changed things around for him completely. You begin to elaborate on how a combination of therapy, antidepressants, and a strong will led him to get back on his feet and become the awesome worker that he once was. Peter will be stirred by this emotional take of will over a challenging situation that was accomplished by seeking the help of a therapist. He will most likely be moved and inspired by the emotional account of an unlikely hero's tale of fighting all odds to emerge victoriously. Of course, you made up or fabricated that entire tale. None of your co-workers or even someone you ever knew had their child slip into a coma, following an accident. There was no depression and no looming fear of a layoff. You just devised that story as a means to manipulate Peter into seeking professional help for his deteriorating psychological condition. It can at best be seen as a way for bypassing a person's defenses or obstinate, where reason or rationale does not seem to work. Manipulation opens that tiny window of hope where you can get your loved ones to do what is good for them.

Well, there's no denying that the strategy you resorted to was manipulative, scheming, dishonest and may be deceptive. However, it was also an innovative, resourceful and creative way to get Peter to do what you wanted him to do for his own well-being. If it leads him to reevaluate or rethink about his own reluctance about seeing a therapist, it may be worth it. In this case, it can be hardly classified as immoral, unethical or unprincipled. You're manipulating your friend into thinking and believing something as someone who cares about him. Sure you may have taken the recourse of devious ways, but your intention was compassionate and unselfish. This is exactly what sets apart negative manipulation from constructive or well-intended manipulation. It is the intention that sets the tone for whether someone is using manipulation in a positive (caring, loving and compassionate) or negative (selfish, deceitful and self-fulfilling) manner.

Plenty of therapists use constructive manipulation for helping their clients transform their lives. Think back to all the instances where you've been slightly imaginative and shifted from a more conventional approach to promote someone else's welfare. You are doing this simply to boost your odds of reaching out to a person who seems shut off to a more straightforward, traditional approach that is linked to his or her own welfare. We use such techniques without even realizing them to minimize another person's resistance and bring about a positive behavioral change.

Sometimes, much like the world leaders, we discussed above, we use constructive manipulation to bring about a beneficial change at a social or human level. This change is good for everyone or the overall good of a family, workplace, community, nationality, race or humanity. Using manipulation to bring about a positive change isn't as devious, evil or crafty as manipulation is made out to be. When straightforward techniques do not work too well in getting people to respond, manipulation proves to be the last ditch attempt.

Much like any other tool or method, nothing is inherently good or bad. Its positivity and negativity lie in the manner in which it is used. C'mon now, even when you are training a puppy to "sit" by holding their favorite treat over their head, aren't you actually manipulating the creature to do what you want them to? Well yes, it is called training you may argue. But that's just clever wordplay or semantics. You are training your puppy, so it leads a more disciplined life that keeps it out of harm. In future, it will find a good home should you have to give it away if it is well trained. So, is manipulating the puppy in such a scenario dubious and evil? No, right?

If you've raised kids or currently fulfilling the herculean task of being a parent, you pretty well know what constructive manipulation is. We are constantly teaching them lessons we want them to believe in. We make up stories about angels, Santa Claus, witches and fairies to get them to do what we want them to for their own welfare. We all know eating vegetables or fruits will not give them superpowers, but sometimes that is the only way to get them to agree to eat it. Several times more subtle or gentle types of manipulation can be utilized for motivating or inspiring people to do things that are more beneficial or safer for them. These approaches can be used to transform a person's self-image. If you are manipulating someone to quit smoking or give up junk food, that isn't such an evil thing, is it? Think of manipulation as fire. It is a powerful, lethal tool that can be used to offer warmth as well as cause destruction. How you choose to use it is totally up to you. It's like that little matchstick you have in your hand. You can light the fireplace or a bunch of candles to keep you and your loved ones cozy and comfortable or you can misuse it to cause devastation.

2. Negative Manipulation.

Negative reinforcement is a form of psychological manipulation which is used to make people feel obligated to act in certain ways in order to avoid certain levels of mental or physical pain or discomfort. In positive reinforcement, you get a reward for acting the way the manipulator wants you to act, and the desire for that reward is what modifies your behavior in the future. Negative reinforcement is, however, a bit more complicated than that. To understand the concept of negative reinforcement, you first have to understand how it's different from punishment. Both of them are popular manipulation techniques, but there is a subtle difference between them. Many people assume that they are the same thing, but they are not. In punishment, the manipulator adds something negative when you don't act a certain way. In negative reinforcement, the manipulator subtracts something negative when you act the way they want you to act. Reinforcement is meant to strengthen voluntary responses, while punishment is meant to weaken voluntary responses; the manipulator will choose one method or the other based on the kind of outcome that they desire in that particular situation.

While punishment is meant to stop a certain behavior from occurring again, reinforcement is meant to encourage the behavior to occur again. A manipulator would use punishment to stop you from doing something he doesn't want you to do. However, he will use negative reinforcement to force you to do (or to keep doing) something he wants. For example, nagging is more of a negative reinforcement technique than a punishment. When someone wants you to do something, they keep nagging you to do it, and the nagging (which is the negative stimulus) stops when you comply. So, negative reinforcement works on you because you want to put a stop to a negative stimulus that already exists, while punishment works because you want to keep something negative from happening. Every time someone does something negative to twist your arm to get you to take a certain course of action; that is negative reinforcement. When you are trying to break up with someone, and he/she cries very loudly about it in a public place, until you change your mind, they are using negative reinforcement to manipulate you (at that moment, you feel that the uncomfortable stares from strangers will only stop if you take the person back).

Sanctions are also a very common form of negative reinforcement. They are used by powerful nations to get other nations to bend to their will, but they can also be used in interpersonal relationships or at work in one form or another. A sanction is basically a threat of a future consequence if you fail to do something. Sanctions may be used in relationships for the common good or for malicious intentions; you have to assess the individual situation to tell if the use of sanctioning (or any other negative reinforcement technique) is malicious. Since childhood, most of us have experienced fear manipulation. Our parents manipulated and controlled us by physical discipline or emotional blackmail, and our teachers managed us by threats and humiliation. Unfortunately, our perspectives and beliefs weren't changed at all, only our behaviors—and those changed only temporarily. What many learned by the time they were teenagers is that they didn't want to be around parents and teachers, and the friends or peers whose realities were similar became our closest network with the greatest amount of influence over them. To illustrate this point, let's look at Raul. Raul entered the tenth-grade with a reputation for being a trouble-maker. He harassed all the girls in class, destroyed the classroom desks and books, and disrespected his teachers. When Raul tried his usual tactics with his English teacher, Miss Slater, she decided to call his father. Expecting that Raul's father would offer his support, she never dreamed he'd come down to the school and humiliate Raul in front of all his friends.

Unfortunately, Raul had to sit next to his father all day long as his father accompanied him to every class, pulling him by the ear from one room to another. Did it put the fear of God in him? I'm sure it did. Unfortunately, when the fear factor no longer held him hostage, Raul's behavior was even more disrespectful and threatening than before. He still harassed the girls in class, but now he warned them if they told he would meet them outside the classroom and make them sorry. What Raul's father had taught him was to manipulate through fear. Because Raul didn't experience positive manipulation, his reality was the same—act out and get all the attention you want. Since negative attention was all the attention Raul every experienced, he knew no better.

Not only did he continue to disrespect the girls in class, but he covertly sabotaged his teachers with practical jokes that were destructive and dangerous. He blew his nose and wiped the discharge between the pages of brand new textbooks. He keyed his teacher's car, and one day he sucked in the fumes from a butane lighter and blew them out as he lighted his breath. The fire was like a torch, catching the girl's hair on fire who sat in front of him. Instead of changing his behavior, practicing manipulation through fear hurt others and got him permanently expelled from school for the remainder of the year.

Comparing Negative Manipulation to Positive Manipulation Attempts.

The next year Raul returned, along with his reputation for being a rebellious bully. By now, his reality was "get them before they get me" school of thought. The fear manipulation hadn't achieved any beneficial changes in Raul's behaviors or perspective, except to reinforce the negative. What made matters worse is he was now a year behind his classmates and in danger of becoming another dropout statistic.

Fortunately for Raul, he got more than he bargained for in one of his new teachers, Mr. Thompson. Mr. Thompson was obviously a teacher who realized how to move and empower his students through positive manipulation; thereby, helping them to create a new reality for themselves. Raul came into the classroom with the same old mean-spirited, sour attitude, but instead of a write-up, after the reprimand, after another write-up, what Raul experienced was a teacher who believed in teaching through the continuous power of healthy relationships. One day, both were in detention—Raul for disciplinary reasons from another hard-nosed teacher, and Mr. Thompson to act as supervisor for after-school detention. Mr. Thompson had a whole week of after-school detention time to build rapport with Raul. Mr. Thompson questioned Raul about his likes and dislikes, only to discover Raul's love for fast cars. Since Mr. Thompson's hobby was rebuilding an old muscle-car he had inherited from his great aunt, he decided to involve Raul in the process. He brought the car to school and stored it in the industrial arts building. Every day after school, Mr. Thompson and Raul would work on the car together.

Through his questions and rapport building, Mr. Thompson manipulated Raul to change his "get them before they get me" perspective on life. The improved behavior that began in Mr. Thompson's class soon spread to other aspects of Raul's life as well. As they finished the car, Mr. Thompson permitted Raul the privilege of taking dates out in his amazing muscle car. Girls had a new respect for Raul and his disrespectful attitude changed for them as well. Raul's mechanical talents surpassed that of Mr. Thompson, and he was often called to the house to assist him with needed repairs, strengthening their friendship and mutual respect.

Although it was a challenge to catch up, Raul passed that year with flying colors. As the years passed, he grew more confident and changed from rebellious to productive. His grades were good, and it was evident Raul had a real talent to repair anything mechanical. Toward the end of his senior year, Raul talked to Mr. Thompson about his inability to afford college and together they discussed other employment options. Graduation night, Raul had the biggest smile of any other student as he collected his diploma, knowing how hard he had worked and how many obstacles he had overcome with Mr. Thompson's help. His mother and father had since divorced, and Raul's mom and younger brother were the only ones who cheered him on that evening. He searched the crowd for Mr. Thompson's familiar cheery face but was disappointed when he failed to see him in the line of teachers wishing their students good luck in their future endeavors. It was difficult for Raul to hid his disappointment as he slowly led his mother and brother down the front steps and out to the parking lot. Raul felt so sorry for himself that he didn't see the bright red, 1965, convertible Mustang GTX at first until his mother touched his arm and spoke in a tearful voice. "Raul, I think Mr. Thompson has a surprise for you."

"I looked for him, but…"

"He's right there with your present."

There parked right in front of the steps was the car they had worked on for two years. It had a huge gold ribbon around it, with the words "Class of 1999" written on the window. Mr. Thompson was there to hand Raul the keys and wish him good luck in his future endeavors.

Chapter 3: Emotional Manipulation

This is not wholly distinct from the carrot and the stick but much of manipulating people involves emotional intelligence. There are a variety of ways in which people emotionally manipulate others. All of these, in some sense, work with the tools above to affect the actions of another. It might seem natural to conclude that the goal of emotional manipulation is to provoke irrational behavior – however, that's rarely the case. Emotional manipulation is much more likely to distort the truth, to the extent that someone's alters their path to achieve their goals, through a perceived change in reality. Examine an approach to emotional manipulation called the guilt trip. The guilt trip involves trying to make someone feel worse about an action they have taken (or an action they have failed to take, which amounts to the same thing i.e. sitting around and not tidying your room is an action).

By guilt tripping someone, you are attempting to affect their emotional reaction to their error. The return is for that person to feel indebted. You are altering their perception of a situation, so that they will either: correct their behavior at the next opportunity or make amends for their error.

Here is a breakdown of the mechanics:

• They are concerned about their loss of reputation. If they develop a reputation as someone who cannot or will not help others to achieve their goals, the result will be a loss of power. Solving the issue by making amends is a way to salvage their reputation.

• You are persuading them of the severity of their error. As previously mentioned, failing deception, this requires you to either offer genuine new information, such as a previously unknown negative impact of their error – perhaps a financial cost to yourself or another – or have enough of their trust that they believe your opinion of opinion of events to be valid, causing them to reassess their own.

• Naturally, you can use deception to fabricate the above – inventing a detail that changes their perspective. An example could be lying about an injury they caused to someone else unintentionally, playing up its severity. While you will be found out eventually, this might be an effective short term tactic to provoke a confession.

• The person who has committed the error is also affected by your power. If you have the ability to remedy the problem they have caused, they are likely to be submissive to your demands. Your power is the ability to help them achieve their goal of saving their reputation and naturally that increases, the greater they perceive their error to be. Guilt tripping is far from the only form of emotional manipulation. It is difficult to draw the line between ethical and unethical emotional manipulation. For example, what constitutes guilt tripping as opposed to simply expressing disappointment? They are essentially the same. Likewise, what is the difference between intimidation and

Fortunately, this book is avoiding these issues for now but you'll find more information on the ethics of manipulation in the next chapter. There are many terms for many different types of emotional manipulation. It is not necessary to memorize, or even learn, all of them. By understanding the mechanics of emotional manipulation, you can easily analyze and understand them as they arise. Here are a few examples:

• Intimidation – Provoking fear in a target, such that they may alter their strategy for achieving their goals. In particular, intimidation that carries a threat of violence can encourage a target to change their course of action in ensuring their own self-preservation (a fairly universal goal). Acting to appease their intimidator is a way for the target to survive, and becomes their future behavior.

Note that there is nothing irrational in the behavior of the target here. Emotional manipulation is not necessarily the provocation of irrational behavior. Bonus points if you recognized that this is hardly distinct from the "stick."

• Seduction – Manipulating a target by presenting them with an object of desire, and withholding it until the target performs an action. The object may be the seducer or some other asset, like money. Scam emails from Nigerian princes work by seducing the target with the prospect of easy money. Sexual seduction may include provoking irrational behavior, based on the promise of endorphins. An alternative way of viewing this is as a persuasion to manipulate the goals of others, prioritizing a sexual encounter above everything else. Seduction revolves around power, as it is presenting and persuading the ability to offer somebody what they want. Bonus points if you recognized that this is hardly distinct from the "carrot."

• Minimization – This is the effort to reduce someone's perspective of an issue, or error you have caused. It may involve any manipulation tools to reduce the magnitude of the issue.

It normally involves persuasion and deception, highlighting or fabricating facts to demonstrate the lack of importance. It can also involve rationalization, which is explaining the reasons for one's actions in an attempt to justify them.

Although this bears no direct relation to power, observe how differently people respond to this behavior from someone who has perceived power, compared to someone who is perceived to lack it.

• Blaming – Passing the blame for an error onto someone else is a way to preserve your power, by protecting your reputation, using either persuasion or deception.

Note how easy it becomes to break down familiar actions, like blaming, using these three tools.

As well as passing the blame, creating blame can also be a useful smokescreen. Blaming a victim is a way of persuading a victim that their reputation is under threat, in order to manipulate a vulnerable person. At this point, you may also recognize that blaming is closely linked to intimidation. There is damage or the threat of damage to someone's reputation, which can alter their actions by making them feel responsible or concerned that others will hold them responsible.

Chapter 4: Covert Manipulation Technique

Covert is when an attempt is made to communicate with the subject's unconscious mind without the subject knowing that he or she will be put through hypnosis. It comprises a string of technique such as conversational hypnosis or NLP (neuro-linguistic programming), body language and other powerful communication and interaction strategies. The primary objective of covert hypnosis is to gradually change an individual's behavior at a subconscious level to lead the subject into believing that they changed their mind on their own accord. You simply lead them into believing that they weren't influencer or manipulated by changed their mind on their own. When covert hypnosis is successfully performed, the subject isn't aware that he or she is being hypnotized. There is considerable debate about the fine line between conventional hypnotism and covert hypnotism. While standard hypnotism is about drawing the focus of the subject, covert hypnotism is primarily about relaxing the subject a bit or softening their stand by using deception, confusion, interruption and a series of other techniques. If you've watched the series "The Mentalist," you'll realize that covert hypnosis is used in a particular instance when a perpetrator tries to influence various characters and tries to murder her employer.

8 Proven Covert Hypnosis Techniques

Here are some forms of covert hypnosis techniques for beginners

1. Deception

Deception is one of the most commonly practiced covert hypnosis techniques to lead the subject into doing what you want without them knowing about your real intentions. For instance, you may want a close friend to give up addiction and resort to plain deception to lead them away from their addiction triggers or suggest something false without making them catch your true intentions of making them give up alcohol or drugs. As a practiced hypnotist, you create an illusion or sense of false reality to help the subject believe something you want them to. We have all been susceptible to deception at some point or the other. There is a tendency of believing fictional information without ever asking for details. Clairvoyants, psychics, and hypnotists used this method generously to create an illusion by gaining the explicit trust of the subject through clever rapport-building techniques.

2. Eye Contact Clues

People almost always display a particular body language type that reflects their deepest thoughts and feelings. Hackneyed as it sounds, "Eyes are truly windows to one's soul." Analyzing an individual's body language (especially their eyes) will award you with a good sense of how a particular word, action, sound, image or emotion is perceived by him or her. The subject is read based the direction's his or her eyes are darting in. Examine the subject's eyes thoroughly for cues.

This technique is more complicated than it sounds and needs plenty of practice.

3. Misdirection

This covert hypnosis technique is widely used by magicians all over the world to manipulate their audience or create an illusion. Magicians sneakily use the power of misdirection to distract their audience's attention to another point of focus to perform a quick action that they wish to hide. For instance, if you are attempting to get the subject to do something by directly sowing the suggestion, they are more consciously aware of your intentions. However, if you are accomplishing the same goal, you distract their attention elsewhere and make the same suggestion worded in another context.

4. Sub modalities

There is great variance between the responses of different to the same information. This can be detected by the manipulator using several sub modalities (under various contexts) to generate the desired response. Look for voice tone, body language, facial expressions and eyes cues. When the use of certain words or actions creates positive submodalities, you can continue using them to invoke specific feelings or emotions.

5. Generalized Reading

Generalized or warm reading is a covert hypnosis technique based on making a generalized observations or statements that could be applicable for just about anyone that do not take into account unique observations or responses gained from the subject. Fortune tellers, psychic and clairvoyants use a lot of this technique to manipulate their clients into believing that the readings are unique to them, when in fact, these are general observations that can be applicable for just about any person.

For instance, "You are an ambitious person who also strives for happiness, contentment and inner peace. You've learned and evolved from your past experiences. You have overcome your past mistakes to look forward to new and exciting life ahead." You can ask any person to read this, and he or she will end up believing this was written only with him or her in mind. It leads the subject's mind to believe that it is about him or her since they are unique. Warm readings can be used as icebreakers to establish a rapport of trust with the subject (by making seemingly accurate statements) before they begin to talk. This gives you the advantage to build upon the all too accurate beginning statement.

6. Hot Reading

Hot reading differs from general or warm readings in a manner that you have some prior information about the subject (which he or she is completely unaware of), which completely amazes them. You've got to find a way to obtain important bits of information about a person without him or knowing about it, which can be tricky. The subject will then be led into believing that you have been blessed with supernatural or psychic abilities.

7. Cold Observations

While warm observations involve making generalized statements that can be applicable to everyone and hot observations are sneakily obtaining specific information about a person to use it to your advantage, cold observations are made based on your initial impression about a person by closely studying them. You then build upon the general statements by making more specific statements based on their responses. It is regularly used by mentalists, psychics, and spiritualists to form an illusion that can accurately read a person's mind or perform telepathy. Subjects are led into believing that they are indeed everything they are told they are by the manipulator. It comprises making vague statements after making a few first impression observations of an individual, which can easily be acquired after practicing a few people reading and analyzing skills. For example, you can simply say to your subject, "I have a feeling you are a self-assured and confident individual although you tend to hesitate at times based on past experiences." You wait for a response from the subject.

The subject can come up with a bunch of responses such as, "yes, you're right. I am generally confident and expressive but tend to be held back by past experiences" (which means they are generally confident people), "Oh yes, I do tend to reflect a lot on my past actions" (which means they are more shy and hesitant than self-assured and confident). Once they respond to a general statement, you can use their response to make more specific or direct statements about the person.

8. Ericksonian Hypnosis Theory

This technique comprises using stories, examples and anecdotes for eliminating the wall of resistance built by our subconscious mind. The hypnotizer or manipulator narrates a story, which ends with a moral that the manipulator desires to convey. The subject's subconscious mind builds a connection or deep relationship with different aspects of the story. You lead the subject into emotionally linking with the story that sounds similar to the situation they are in currently. This is s strategy for making indirect suggestions using a story to distract or divert the conscious mind, thus leaving the unconscious more receptive to suggestions.

Chapter 5: NLP Manipulation Techniques

NLP or Neuro Linguistic Programming is one of today's most widely used mind control, persuasion, manipulation and influencing techniques. It is applied by everyone from salespersons to political leaders to media bigwigs. The method was invented by John Grinder and Richard Bandler in the 70s, and its popularity spiraled in the world of marketing, public relations, advertising, sales and even personal/social relationships. People who master NLP are known to be equipped with the ability to trick people into doing whatever they want them to in several incredible ways. The duo Bandler and Grinder came up with a sort of new age version of hypnotherapy. While conventional hypnosis is dependent upon putting the subject or client into a state of trance, NLP isn't as heavily loaded. It is about layering or planting suggestions into the subject's unconscious mind through the clever use of language or semantics, without them knowing that you are using the technique.

Today the strategies of NLP and hypnotic writing are widely used in the internet marketing, social media and make money online scams. The sales copy of most get rich quick schemes is cleverly worded to manipulate the unsuspecting reader into taking the intended action. People trained in the art of NLP are experts in watching out for eye movements, pupil dilation, flush of the skin and other neurologically linked signals that reveal plenty about the person's thought process.

For instance, simply by observing a person an NLP trained person can determine what side of the brain is dominantly used by the individual. They can also identify what sense (sight, hearing, smell, etc.) is most powerful in the person. The manner in which the brain organizes, stores and uses information (can be determined through a person's eye movements) and when they are giving false information or making stories.

For example, an individual who is primarily focused on seeing will use words and phrases that hold visual metaphors such as, "Do you really see my point?" Similarly, a person is more focused on hearing with tend to use "Hear me" or "I hear you." This is the language that you should stick to as a manipulator trying to get them to do what you want. You'll score higher points with a visual person by using words such as "look at the situation in this way." It is all about wording your talks in a way that plays on their linguistic programming. By mirroring a person's body language and specific linguistic patterns, the manipulator is aiming to build a rapport. It is a psychological process where a person lets their guard down and arrives at the conclusion that the manipulator or NLPer is similar to them or like them. What the NLPer does is fakes certain social clues that lead a person to drop the defenses they build around themselves for other people (especially strangers). This makes them more open and receptive to any suggestions that the NLPer plans to embed in their mind.

NLP helps the manipulator train others into thinking and doing what they want. It is about influencing the subject's thoughts, feelings, and behavior in a way that is beneficial for the manipulator. Skilled manipulators know how to use the power of anchors (external influences) for sparking or triggering specific emotions in people. For instance, a song that is associated with the subject's first kiss can be used for triggering all emotions related to that moment.

Do not we all experience this in everyday life? Certain songs remind us of particular moments or phases in our life and hence become associated with the emotions we felt during those moments or phases. Each time we hear those songs, our subconscious experiences the same feelings and emotions. The song in this example acts as the emotional anchor to help induce feelings and emotions that you want in the other person.

Let's take another example. Each time a person buys coffee for you, you talk about something pleasant that happened in his or her life like his or her marriage or the birth of his child. If you talk about the birth of his or her child consistently every time the person buys you coffee, they will come to associate buying coffee for you with pleasant, positive emotions. It acts as a sort of anchor for his or her feelings. NLP is a complex discipline that cannot be acquired in a day. It needs hours and hours of practice with reading people's subconscious behavior, understanding their neurological programming and more. However, as beginner manipulator, you'd want to understand some popular techniques used by NLPers on their subjects.

Here are a few expert techniques NLPers use to manipulate people or control their minds.

1. They Observe Eye Movements

NLPers will always closely observe their subject's eye movements to determine what part of the brain is being used, and how the subject stores/uses information. They give the impression that they are keenly interested in what the other person is saying and actually care about knowing their thoughts when in reality they are simply analyzing how a person access information from different parts of his or her brain. Within a few minutes, practitioners of NLP can tell if a person is lying or telling the truth. The subject will almost end up believing that the manipulator has some psychic abilities or telepathic superpowers. NLPers carefully calibrate eye movements to know conclude which parts of a brain are most active in a person, and how they process information.

2. Use the Power of Touch

NLPers use the power of touch effectively to induce certain feelings and emotions in their subjects without the subject even realizing it. Let us say for instance that the subject is in a particular state of emotion such as happy, angry, upset, sad, etc., NLP practitioners will use touch (light tap on the subject's shoulder or touch their arm) and anchor that particular form of touch by linking it to a specific emotion. Each time you want to invoke that specific emotion in a person to fulfill your intent, simply use the particular touch that you did when the subject was experiencing the same emotion earlier.

3. Use Vague Words and Phrases

One of the fundamental methods of NLP is the generous use of vague verbiage for inducing a sort of hypnotic trance on the subject. NLPers believe that the more ambiguous and vague your language, the less likely is to your subject to opposing your ideas or disagree with you, thus making it easier to lead them into the trance state. You are basically limiting their ability to react to what you are saying. Did you notice how effectively former United States of America President Barrack Obama used this technique during the famous "change campaign?" It was a word wrought in complete ambiguity. Anyone could interpret it in a way they wanted.

4. Relaxed and Permissive Words

Expert NLP hypnotists never start by telling their subjects what they want them to do outright. The commands follow more permissive and relaxed issuances such as "please feel free to de-stress or relax" or "you can have this for as long as you like" or "you're welcome to test this product." The subject is sort of given a loose rope, and the impression that the NLPer really wants to relax and enjoy without restrictions. The language use is more relaxing and permissive. Skilled hypnotists realize that this is more effective when it comes to driving the subject into a state of trance over immediately commanding them into it. When you begin with, "please feel free to let your hair down and relax completely", they are likelier to go into a trance gradually.

5. Layered Language

Skilled NLPers will always use language that is deeply layered or has hidden meaning/connotations attached to it. They'll use widely believed facts and slowly slip in their agenda into to manipulate the subject's subconscious mind into thinking in a particular way. For example, food, sleep and going outdoors with me are the formula for a healthy life. On the surface of it, the subject's subconscious mind tends to agree with it because everyone has been conditioned to believe that food, sleep and getting fresh air is good for their health. They will tend to agree with it without giving it much thought. However, the layered message here is – going outdoors with me. And boy did you just get someone to agree to that on a subconscious level? This is an extremely subtle yet powerful NLP technique that is harnessed to the hilt by experienced NLP practitioners.

You also follow up one question with another to create what can be termed as a conditioning by association. For example, you ask someone, "How many fingers are there on the human hands?" followed quickly by "How many on ten hands?" The answer to the first will be ten, while the answer to the second question most likely will be 100. The first is, of course, right, while the second is wrong. The answer to the second is 50. As an NLPer, you are creating a trap for getting your subject to think the way you want to through careful conditioning through association. In NLP, you essentially build anchors or baselines that you can lead your subjects to whenever you want. It can come to anyone with a little bit of training and practice.

Talking about the power of association, it is widely used by advertisers to manipulate consumers into associating certain products with specific attributes and lifestyles. For instance, Coca-Cola always has these fancy advertisements about beautiful young people gulping glasses of bottles of the aerated beverage. They are hot (or cool if you please), rich, in gorgeous settings and look extremely cheerful. What are your impressions as you consume those images? That drinking Coca-Cola gives you access to the good life. The idea and associations are deeply installed and embedded in the subconscious mind and leads you to make a rather quick decision when it comes to purchasing.

6. Get them to Agree

If you can get your subjects to answer in the affirmative to several questions in a row, it will be tough for them to refuse your final request. NLPers know this only too well and use it liberally on their subjects to get them to do what they want. This is one of the many clever manipulation and persuasion strategies used by sales and marketing folks. They will launch into a series of questions, the answer of which will rarely ever be in negative. After getting consecutive positive replies from their subjects, they will go for the kill and lead them into making impulsive and emotionally driven decisions. The entire technique is designed for engineering spur of the moment decisions by switching off the subject's ability to make logical decisions.

For example, an insurance salesperson will ask his client questions such as

"Wouldn't you like to financially secure the future of your loved ones?" Yes. "Wouldn't you like to use a policy that offers hassle-free claims?" Yes.

"Wouldn't you want to protect your family's dream for a low as \$123/month?" Yes. "Wouldn't you like your children's education and future dreams taken care of even when you aren't around?" Yes. "Wouldn't you want coverage for the immediate family under one policy at a single rate?" Yes.

"Then you should not waste any more time because you never know what happens in the next moment. Sign up for the policy immediately while it is available for a low monthly premium for a limited period."

See how a person is led into making a decision using the power of affirmatives or getting someone to agree to a series of questions before finally getting them to agree to the main thing. This can be as effective when you're asking someone out on a date. When a person replies in the affirmative to a series of mostly emotional questions posed by the NLPer, it is hard for the subject to refuse the final offer.

7. Use Gibberish

NLP practitioners resort to using a lot of gibberish mumbo-jumbo with the intention of attempting to program the subjects internal emotions and leading them into where the manipulator wants them to go. As an NLPer, you can't afford to be specific or explain precisely what you meant. You have to utilize trance invoking ambiguous language that throws the subject off gear and allows you to take complete control of their feelings and emotions. Phrases such as, "As you let go of this emotion slowly, you will see yourself transitioning into a state of alignment with the aura of your success." It does not make any sense in the logical scheme of things, but your subject is befuddled into doing exactly what you want him or her to. Since it cannot be comprehended immediately, they'll be less prone to rejecting it in a state of confusion. When you do not know what to do or can't think for yourself, you are more susceptible to blindly following the instructions of the person who is guiding or leading you.

Chapter 6: Dark Psychology

Dark Psychology is one of the arts of persuasion and mind control. Psychology refers to the study of the behaviors of human beings. It is the center of every human being's thinking, their deeds, and socialization. Therefore, Dark Psychology is basically the phenomenon through which human beings apply manipulation, persuasion, and mind control techniques to fulfill their intentions. In dark psychology, there is the 'Dark Psychology Triad' which is one of the easiest predictors of manipulator's behavior, collapsed relationships, and also being problematic. The Dark Psychology Triad includes:

• The psychopathy - They are friendly and always charming, impulsive, selfish, lack empathy, and are not remorseful.

• The narcissists - These kinds of people are filled with ego, grandiosity, and have no empathy or sympathy.

• The Machiavellians - These kinds of people use manipulation, persuasion, and mind control to exploit and lure people. In addition to this, they are always immoral.

No one in this world would wish to be a victim of manipulation even though it happens whether you are conscious or unconscious of it. In the case you fall under manipulation, it is not necessarily someone in the Dark Psychology Triad, but you will face persuasion on a daily basis. Manipulation tactics always manifest themselves in regular commercials, Internet advertisements, sales tactics, and in your workplaces. If you are a parent, you must have come across these tactics in your everyday life since children tend to experiment with tactics so that they can get what they want. Dark Psychology is used by people who you genuinely love or trust. In Dark Psychology, the manipulators use the following tactics:

• They flood their targets with love, compliments, and buttering up to acquire what they want.

• They lie too much, exaggerate things, tell untruths or even tell partially true stories.

• They deny their love to those they are targeting through withholding their attention.

• They give some choice routes that distract you from the choice you do not want them to make.

• They apply reverse Psychology, which involves doing something which motivates their victim to do the opposite, which turns out to be what they wanted.

• They use words assumed to have the same definition, but later tell you they meant something else throughout the conversation.

Dark Psychology aims at reminding you how easy it is to get manipulated. You should, therefore, assess your techniques in all areas of your life, workplace, leadership, intimate relationships, and parenting. The people who use these Dark Psychology tactics are aware of what they are doing and manipulate you intentionally to get what they want. Some end up using unethical ways in their manipulative techniques though they are never aware of it. Other people learned their manipulative techniques at very early ages. For instance, if you applied a particular behavior when you were a kid, and you got what you wanted, you are more likely to use the same technique every time you want something.

Others are trained or get to know these tactics just by happenstance. The training programs that can prepare you on the ideas and concepts of Dark Psychology and unethical persuasion techniques are mostly the sales and marketing programs. When doing sales or marketing, dark tactics are applied to either create a brand or sell a product which ends up benefiting the sales assistants rather than the customer's needs. You get convinced that using such dark tactics is okay as it helps the buyer. The following are the people who use Dark Psychology tactics the most:

• The Narcissists – Narcissistic people always have a high sense of self-worth. They want everyone to realize and recognize their superiority.

They still want to be adored or worshipped. Therefore, they use dark tactics to manipulate, persuade, or control the minds of their targets.

• The Sociopaths – They are charming, bright, but impulsive. They lack emotions and are remorselessness hence end up using Dark Psychology tactics to mend relationships with people they can easily take advantage of.

• The Attorneys - Most of the attorneys emphasize on winning their cases such that they opt for dark manipulation tactics to acquire what they want.

• Political Figures – They are always using shady manipulation tactics while campaigning for people to elect them. They use dark psychological techniques to prove to the voters that they are the best and deserve the post they are fighting for.

• Salespeople – The salespeople are always focusing on the benefits rather than the customer's satisfaction. They use dark persuasion tactics to make the buyer buy their products.

• Leaders – They use dark manipulation tactics to have great efforts, submission, and higher performance from their dependents.

• Speakers – Various speakers, especially public speakers, practice dark persuasion tactics to influence their audience. This helps them sell more products, predominantly in the final stages.

• The Selfish – Anyone with a hidden agenda of self before others always uses dark manipulation tactics to get what they want first at someone's costs.

Most of Dark Psychology tactics seem to step even on your own toes. Speakers and salespeople are everyday users of these dark tactics. You should, therefore, note that, whether working, writing, talking, or making sales, you are neither supposed to use these dark tactics. Various people tend to admit that their professions require them to practice dark tactics, especially if their aim is maintaining the company's top positions or to avoid losing customers.

It is unfortunate because if they fail to exercise these tactics, there will be short-term sales as well as revenue that will ultimately lead to customers not trusting the company, poor business tactics, employees becoming disloyal, and less successful business results. This calls for you to know the difference between motivation and manipulation tactics that are good or dark. This can be achieved if you assess your intents. If a tactic benefits you alone, then it must be an ominous manipulation task.

How to Use Dark Psychology Techniques Ethically

At Place of work: The three personality characters of the Dark Triad can as well be used ethically at your place of work. It can be used in getting the top leadership positions. You can use your manipulative techniques to have interpersonal influence that can get you promoted easily in your workplace. Internet elves: Most of the people who troll others on the Internet mostly use dark psychology tactics. They are always antisocial, psychopaths, and aggressive. Everyday trolls indicate that people have bad lives behind the keyboards and such has been linked to bullying evident amongst the youths and young adults. As a coupling scheme: Most of the couples use dark triad tactics, primarily in their sex lives. Most people with these personalities steal bedmates from other people and have low self-esteem. Outward Look: At first sight, you can tell a person with dark triad personalities due to their appealing appearance. They concentrate more on their clothing and makeups, a look that could be put down if someone pulled off their clothing and wiped off the makeup. Most of those who concentrate on looks are the narcissists.

Chapter 7: Analysis Techniques

Now that you are clear on why analysis is used and why it is so essential to your manipulation practice, it is time for you to learn how you can actually analyze people! In this chapter, you are going to learn about three primary types of analysis, as well as when you can use them and how you can maintain your secrecy in the process. The three main strategies we are going to pay attention to are: body language (including facial expressions), profiling, and verbal cues. These three areas are the most important when it comes to analyzing someone prior to manipulation.

Body Language

There are two types of body language that you want to pay attention to when you are reading someone's physical expressions: their actual body language, and their facial expressions. Both of these will give you a large amount of insight as to what they are thinking and how they are feeling at any given time.

You want to begin by paying attention to someone's body language before you even begin talking to them. Get a sense of how they carry themselves, how they tend to move and express themselves when different types of things are said to them, and how their body language changes when different moods are experienced. Ideally, the longer you can comfortably observe someone from a distance, the better. This gives you a chance to get a stronger idea of who they are and what they are like before you enter a conversation with them. However, there are many times that you do not get a significantly long period of time to analyze someone before you begin your conversation. In these circumstances, it is beneficial to have already spent time practicing analyzing people and then use this practice to generate an idea of how your target is feeling and their personality in a short amount of time.

When you are reading someone's body language, start by getting a "baseline" of what they are normally like. Pay attention to their face, their arms and hands, and their feet. Also, if they are walking, notice their gait and how quickly or slowly they are walking. You also want to know how they are carrying themselves. Then, once you get a baseline, take a moment to pay attention to how their baseline changes with different stimulus. For example, when they are happy or when they are annoyed. You want to essentially get an idea of their three primary states that matter most to you: normal, positive, and negative. This will help you when it comes to conversing, as it will give you an idea of whether they are having a positive or negative reaction to what you are saying to them.

The benefit of body language is that virtually everyone has a similar type of body language expression. This is a form of communication that we unknowingly learn as we grow up, and because we all tend to communicate in the same way, our body language tends to work in the same way from person to person. For this reason, if you do not have a long time to observe or analyze someone first, you can use basic body language knowledge to generate an idea of what they are thinking and feeling, and about how they are feeling in response to various things you say or offer them. Now that you understand body language and how you should be reading it, let's start focusing on specific cues and readings that you can understand from someone when you are analyzing them. In the following sections we are going to explore three types of body language: the body language itself, walking or mobile body language, and facial expressions.

Body Language

Body language comes in two forms: basic cues, and complex cues. Basic cues are ones that you are likely already familiar with. They include ones such as stomping your feet or making fists with your hands when you are angry, slouching in your chair and resting your head in your hands when you are bored or upset about something, and other similar cues. You are likely already familiar with the majority of basic body language cues, so we are going to focus more on the in-depth cues here. Complex body language are things we unconsciously do any time we are feeling a certain way. These cues give on-lookers the ability to know exactly how we are feeling. Most people looking at us only know subconsciously and get a "feeling" about how we are feeling, or they may even overlook it entirely in favor of their own thoughts and feelings. As an experienced body language reader, however, you would be able to easily identify what these cues mean and how they relate to what the person is thinking at any given time. Let's take a look at them, now. When you are reading body language, you typically want to start with getting an idea for a person's overall body language. This is how they tend to carry themselves when they are "at rest" in the conversation. It may vary from conversation to conversation depending on their pre-existing emotions at any given time, but in general you should notice that most people have a fairly neutral "starting" position. Knowing what someone tends to look like when they are in neutral allows you to recognize when they make changes and what these changes mean about how they are feeling and what they are thinking.

To read someone's complex body language, start by looking at their hands and arms. Where are they placed, and what are they doing? Are they near the body, or further away? In general, the further the hands are from the body, the more relaxed a person is feeling. This is true unless the hands are tucked in neatly but are completely relaxed and not tensing, fidgeting, or grasping at anything. If their hand is rested comfortably on their lap, for example, it would show that the person somewhat submissive and relaxed. If both of their hands were folded and rested in the center of their lap, it would show that they were completely submissive in the situation. When people touch their arms with opposing hands, this often signifies that they are feeling uncomfortable or uncertain in a situation and that they are trying to understand it at a greater level. If both hands are touching the opposing arms, however, this indicates that they are feeling shut down on some level. If the hands are relaxed on the opposing arms, the person is feeling defeated. If they are tense, the person is feeling agitated. Sometimes, hands may not be positioned on the body itself at all. Instead, they may be placed elsewhere. For example, on an object. The message then comes from whatever that object is and the tension of the grip on that object. For example, if they are lightly gripping their cup in front of them, they are relaxed but waiting for an appropriate moment to take a drink. If they are holding their purse or keys in their hand, they are ready to leave but are waiting for the right time to say that they are ready to go. If their hands never left their purse or keys, it means they were not intending to stay long and that they may be uncomfortable or untrusting in their surroundings. With hands, there are two things you are looking for: placement, and grip. If the hands are placed on an object, consider what that object means to them. If the object is something that the person would typically use if they stay around for a while, then the person is likely relaxed and well-engaged in their environment. If they are gripping anything such as their keys, their purse, their wallet, the door handle, or otherwise, this means that they are ready to go and do not want to be here any longer. The next place you want to look is at their legs and their feet. Unlike the hands, feet do not grip anything. For that reason, the biggest thing you can learn about someone from their feet comes from which direction the feet are pointing and what movements they are making, if any. Where the feet are pointing says a great deal about what the person is thinking and where they want to go. If, for example, they are pointed at the person in front of them and at the door, that means that they want to leave with that person. If both are pointed at the person, they are comfortable in the environment and completely tuned in to that single person. If they are pointing at multiple people in the conversation, they are engaged in a group conversation. If they are pointing at the bar, they want another drink. If both are pointing at the door, they really want to leave.

The feet may be making a variety of different movements, too. If they are still, this means that the person is either relaxed or focused. They are engaged in whatever is going on around them, and so they are not thinking about any movements. When they begin to move, however, they can signify a variety of things. For example, if a person is feeling anxious, they may rapidly move their feet back and forth. If the feet are only gently rocking back and forth, or if you are looking at a woman and she is slipping the back of her shoe on and off, it means that they are feeling some form of attraction for the person that they are talking to. If a person has their feet crossed at the ankles and they are bouncing them around, this may signify that they are bored and wish that they were somewhere else, or doing something else.

Pay attention to both the hands and the feet when you are reading someone's body language. Both will give you a clear identifying factor of how they are feeling and what they are thinking. The best way to get a full read on a person is to read what both parts of the body are telling you and then put it together as a full message. That way, you know exactly what the person is thinking and feeling.

Walking Cues

How people walk says a lot about how they are feeling in any given moment. In general, the faster they are walking, the less they are thinking. This doesn't necessarily mean that they aren't thinking about anything it all. Instead, it usually means that they are only thinking about one thing. For example, they may be late and they are thinking about what they are late for and so they are walking fast. Or, they may be angry and looking for the person they are upset with, and the only thing on their mind is that anger. Since the faster a person walks translates to less thoughts on a person's mind, the slower a person walks translates to more thoughts on a person's mind. Therefore, if you see someone walking about slowly, they are often thinking about a lot. They may be walking slowly with an inquisitive look on their face, as though they are pondering something large and looking for the answer while they walk. Or, they may be walking slowly with a somewhat dazed look on their face, thinking about anything that comes to their mind.

Aside from the speed of a person's walk, think about their posture, too. A person who walks with a tall, straight back and their head held high is one who is confident and sure of themselves. Someone who walks with their shoulders slumped down and their back shrugged forward and barely picks up their feet is someone who is feeling unconfident. If a person generally walks with a tall, straight posture, and you see them walking with a shrunken, slumped posture, this likely means that they are upset about something in the moment. If the opposite happens, then the person is likely happy and has experienced some form of achievement in the very recent past. In general, the taller and straighter someone's posture is when they are walking, the surer of themselves they are. This can go all the way up to them having their chin turned upwards as they look down their nose at people, meaning that they likely have a grandiose sense of self-worth. Likewise, the more shrunken and slumped their posture is, the less sure they are of themselves. This goes all the way down to being completely slumped and skulking along, showing that they are feeling really low and down on their luck.

Facial Expressions

There are three areas you want to pay attention to one someone's face when you are using it as a tool for analysis. These three areas include the mouth, cheeks, and eyebrows. These three parts of the face have the tendency to move the most when it comes to expressive looks, and therefore they will also tell you the most about what a person is thinking or feeling at any given time. Facial expressions change rapidly throughout conversations, so pay close attention to these. In general, an emotion will first be expressed on the face, then into the body. They say that if a negative emotion is already being expressed in the body, it's too late and you may have lost the trust and faith of your target when it comes to manipulation. You have to be very swift and confident to turn that emotion around and regain their attention and trust.

With the mouth, there are many things you can tell. For example, someone who's mouth is soft and relaxed is either bored or uninterested in what you are presently talking about. You are losing their attention, and fast. If their mouth is slightly pursed, this is usually the sign that the person is interested in what you are saying and that you have their focus. If the mouth is tightly pursed or even pushed out slightly, this would indicate that they are angry and trying to "bite their tongue" from what they want to say. Smiling typically indicates happiness, but smiling with soft eyes that do not feature crow's feet at the sides indicates that the smile may be out of nervousness or obligation. A true smile always results in the eyes crunching and expressing crow's feet at the sides. If someone's mouth is pulled down at the sides, it may indicate they are sad. However, if it is pulled down and tense in any way, it may instead indicate defensiveness or annoyance. The biggest thing to pay attention for in someone's cheeks is their tension. If someone's cheeks are tight and pulled back towards the ears, this typically indicates that the person is feeling fearful or nervous. If they are tight and pushed forward toward the mouth, this would mean that the person is feeling angry. If the person's cheeks are tight and pressed up toward the eyes, this would indicate that the person is feeling happy. If they are soft or seem to be drooping toward the floor, this would indicate that the person is feeling sad.

Lastly, the eyebrows are another expressive place on the face that you need to pay attention to. If a person's eyebrows are pulled down at the edges and turned upward slightly in the center, this would indicate that they are feeling sad or even pitiful. If they are furrowed, this would mean that they are focusing and trying to take everything in. However, if they furrow and their entire face tenses up, this would indicate that they are angry.

Eyebrows that stay lightly raised for the entire conversation indicate that the person is interested in what you are talking about. However, eyebrows that quickly flicker up and then down indicate that a person is surprised by a piece of information. If they are fairly neutral and don't move, this means the person may be disinterested.

Profiling

Profiling is where you look at someone's surroundings to get a better idea of who they are. This can be easy in some cases, and harder in others. Let's take a look at the three main areas you want to pay attention to with profiling: who they are with, what they look like, and their environment.

Who Are They with?

Start with who the person is with. If the person is close with the person or people they have come in with, then the interactions you see between those two people will be more accurate to how that person feels when they are comfortable. It also allows you to look at the pair or group as a whole to get a feel for what they are like. For example, if they are all dressed in a country-esque theme, you can conclude that they may be more outdoorsy and do-it-yourself type people. However, if they are all dressed in business or business casual clothes, their preferences may lean more toward outsourcing things and getting the best of the best - already made for them. If they are with people they are not typically with, you will be able to tell as the interactions will be a little tenser between them. Although they may still be comfortable, especially if the person is confident, it may seem a little more professional than casual, even if they aren't together for anything business-related.

What Do They Look Like?

Pay attention specifically to what the person you are targeting looks like. Are they well-groomed? Do they look after themselves well? Or are they unkempt and looking somewhat messy? This can give you an idea of how they feel about themselves, and how they think others feel about them, too. If they are well-dressed and groomed, this would indicate that they are confident and care what other people think and want to be perceived well by others. If they are unkempt and not well groomed, it may indicate that they feel low on self-esteem and self-confidence and that they don't overly care about what other people think of them because they don't think that they are worth high praise in the first place. In addition, pay attention to what they are wearing. Their sense of style will tell you a lot about who they are. Bold, bright clothes that have fancy designs, for example, indicate that a person's personality would be bold, bright, and unique. If their clothes are boxy, unfitted, and dull, however, the person may lack individuality and not have a clear sense of who they are. Someone who dresses neatly and in neutral colors likely believes everything should be clean-cut and modern, and has a fairly similar clean-cut personality to match it.

What is Their Environment?

Lastly, pay attention to their environment. The places they spend the most of their time equate to the places they feel most comfortable in. If they're spending a lot of time at concerts and at friend's houses, this would clearly indicate that they are outgoing and into a party lifestyle. If they are regularly spending time at up-scale bars, high end fashion boutiques and galas, this would indicate that they are a part of "high society" and that they like things to be the best of the best. If you can, pay attention to their home, or how they keep their work space and car, too. If they keep them clean and organized, this indicates that the person is someone who has a clear frame of mind and works best in a clear and organized space. If they keep things messy and chaotic, it likely reflects on a disorganized frame of mind and an uncertainty about things. They are also less likely to be reliable than those who are more clean and organized.

Chapter 8: Manipulation Techniques

Everyone in the world has likely used manipulation at some points in their lives. This could have been through telling the most straightforward lies to get out of situations or by flirting with others to get what you want. In understanding the techniques used by manipulators in their work, you need to ask yourself the following question:

Who is at threat from a manipulator? To regulate their victims, the pullers of the strings (manipulators) use several tactics, but most importantly, they do this by targeting specific kinds of personalities. You are more likely to be a victim of manipulation if you have low self-esteem, if you are inexperienced, pleased easily, if you are not confident about yourself and if you lack assertive instincts.

What are the requirements for successful manipulation? Primarily, successful manipulation encompasses a manipulator. Manipulation is also likely to be achieved through covert hostile methods. For successful persuasion, a manipulator has to:

• Cover their violent purposes, deeds, and be friendly.

• Be aware of the psychological susceptibilities of the targeted person so as to conclude which strategies are likely to be the most effective.

• Have an adequate level of callousness to have no doubts about triggering injury to the victim if necessary.

The manipulators exploit different defenselessness habits that exist in the victim's character and such include:

• The naïveté of the targeted person - Based on naïveté, the targeted person experiences hardships to buy the notion that many human beings are always sneaky, deceitful, and hard-nosed. This means if you are the victim, you will be in denial that you are being victimized.

• If you are over-conscientiousness - This is where you find yourself ready to grant the exploiter the advantage of distrust. The manipulator ends up blaming you and supporting their side, which makes you trust them easily. If you are too honest, you end up thinking everyone else is reliable as well.

• Self-confidence - Controllers often check whether you are a self-doubting person and whether you lack self-assertiveness, and this makes you go into a defensive mode effortlessly. You end up not giving a second thought about errors.

• Over-intellectualization - This makes it hard for you to understand and therefore, you end up believing your manipulator's reasons for being hurtful.

• Your emotional reliance - If you have a submissive personality, you are more likely to be a victim of manipulation. The more you rely on your emotions, the more vulnerable you are to being manipulated.

• Loneliness - If you are a lonely person, you are likely to agree to take little proposals of social interaction. Some manipulators will propose being your companion, but at a price. This also involves being narcissistic whereby, you fall easily for any kind of unjustified flattery. Lonely people act without any consultations. Therefore, loneliness goes hand in hand with being impulsive.

• Materialistic - Having a get-rich-quick mindset makes you cheap prey for manipulators. This means you are greedy and want to get rich quickly, hence end up acting immorally for some sort of material exchange.

• The elderly are also at a higher risk of getting controlled easily because they are fatigued and not able to multitask. Likelihoods the elderly will have a thought that a manipulator might be a conman are very rare. Manipulators thus take advantage of them and commit elder abuse.

Techniques of Manipulation

Manipulators take time to explore and examine your characteristics and find out how vulnerable you are to exploitation. They tend to control their victims by playing with their psychological characters. Having read the points above, now you need to know what the tactics and techniques are manipulators use to control their victims. They include various methods, as discussed below.

Techniques of manipulation

Reinforcement: This can be either positive, negative, or intermittent forms of reinforcement.

1 Positive reinforcement: This involves the case where the manipulator uses praises, charms, crocodile tears, unnecessary apologizing, public acknowledgment, cash, presents, consideration, and facial languages like forced laughter or smiles.

2 Negative reinforcement: A manipulator removes you from a negative situation as a favor.

3   Intermittent reinforcement: This is also known as partial reinforcement. This creates an environment full of fear and doubts. It encourages the victim of manipulation to persist.

Punishment: The manipulator acts in a nagging manner. There is yelling, silent treatment, intimidating behavior, and threatening of the victim. Manipulators cry and tend to play the victim card, thus emotionally blackmailing the victim and can go further by swearing they are the innocent one.

Lying: it entails two ways; lying by commission and lying by omission.

1. Lying by commission - You will find it hard to tell when a manipulator is lying the moment they do it, and the truth won't reveal itself until it is too late. You should understand that some people are experts at lying and thus you should not give in easily to their tactics.

2. Lying by omission - This is a subtle way used to manipulate, and it entails telling lies, and at the same time, withholding significant amounts of the facts. It is also applied in propaganda.

Denial: Manipulators rarely admit they are wrong. Even when they have done something wrong, they will refuse to believe it. They are rational and always assert that their behavior is not harmful or they are not as bad as someone else has explained. They accompany every exploitation with phrases like, 'it was only a joke'.

Attention: This includes selective inattention and attention. In this case, manipulators deliberately refuse to listen or pay attention to anything that distracts them from their agendas. They always defend themselves with phrases like, 'I do not need to listen to that'.

Deviation: Controllers never answer any questions directly and always steer the discussion to another topic. If not so, the manipulator gives irrelevant or rogue answers to the direct questions asked.

Intimidation: In this case, the manipulator applies two methods of intimidation; covert intimidation and guilt trip. In underground extortion, the manipulators throw their targets onto the self-justifying side through the use of implied threats. A guilt trip is a technique where the manipulator tries to suggest to the meticulous prey that they no longer care and this makes the victim feel bad and they start doubting themselves, hence, they find themselves in a submissive position.

Use of Sarcasm: The manipulator shames the victim by using put-downs and sarcasm that makes the victim doubt themselves. Making the victim feel unworthy gives an entry for the manipulator to defer the victim. These shaming tactics may include fierce glances, unpleasant tones, rhetorical comments or questions, and subtle sarcasm. Some of the victims end up not daring to challenge the manipulator as it fosters a sagacity of meagerness to their targets. Belittling their Target: Manipulators use this technique to put their target on the self-justifying side, while at the same time, covering the belligerent aims of the persuader. The persuader then misleadingly blames their target in response to the victim's defensive mechanisms. This also involves the case where a manipulator plays the victim role by portraying themselves as victims of circumstances to gain sympathy, thereby, getting what they want. This technique aims at the caring and compassionate victims as they cannot stand seeing someone suffer, and thus, the manipulator takes that chance to get the victim's cooperation.

Feigning: Manipulator pretends that any harm caused was unintentional or they are being accused falsely. Manipulators often wear a surprised face, hence making the victim question their own sanity. Feigning also involves the case where the manipulator plays dumb and pretends they are totally unaware of what the victim is talking about. The victim starts doubting themselves while the manipulator continues to point out the main ideas they included just in case there is any doubt. This happens only if the manipulator had used cohorts in advance that helps them in backing up their stories.

Seduction: In this case, the manipulator uses praise or any form of flattery, which involves supporting the victim to gain their conviction. Manipulators can even start helping you to increase your loyalty, and it will be hard for you to suspect their ill intents. The manipulator can as well play the servant role where their actions will be justified by phrases such as, 'I am just doing my job' or 'I am in service to a certain authority figure.' In this case, the victim will give their trust and end up being manipulated.

Brandishing anger: The manipulator shows off how angry they are in order to intensify the victim's shock to get their submission. In the real sense, the manipulator is never angry, but they act like they are, especially when denied access to what they want. A manipulator can as well control their anger to avoid any confrontations or hide their intents. Manipulators often threaten the victims by saying they are going to report the cases to the police. Anger is a way of blackmailing the victim to avoid telling the truth, as it wards off any further inquiries. This makes the victim focus more on the anger of the manipulator rather than on the manipulation technique being used.

The Bandwagon effect: This is the case where the manipulator tends to comfort the victim by claiming that, whether right or wrong, many people have already done some things, and thus, the victim should do it anyway. The manipulator uses phrases like 'Many people like you...' This kind of manipulation is mainly applied to those under peer pressure conditions. Similar cases are when a manipulator tries to lure the victim into taking drugs or abusing other substances. The techniques discussed above are the tested and proven tactics that any manipulator will strive to use to get a strong control of their victims. Before a manipulator persuades their victims, there are those steps they have to follow to make sure they fully control their victim's minds.

Whatever the reasons for manipulating someone, you should always play your cards safely. That is why you should learn how to manage and control the thoughts of people, the strategies, and steps you need to use in various situations. There are three authentic manipulating skills you can learn quickly through the steps discussed below. If you want to manipulate others in an easy way, come on! Shed a fake tear and follow the following steps.

Effective Steps of Manipulation

Honing Your Persuasion Skills

I. Take an Acting Class: If you want to be a manipulator, you first need to learn how to master your emotions and make others interested in your forced feelings. Now, if you desire to look more distressed that you really are or even want to apply a variety of emotional techniques to get what you want, then take an acting class since it will improve your persuasion powers. When considering an acting class, you need to note you should never tell people you are taking a drama class if you are learning how to persuade and control people's minds. This is because they may get suspicious over your skills rather than believing in you.

II. Taking a Debate Class: After you have taken acting classes and learned how to master your emotions when convincing others to get what you want, you need to take debate classes, which might also involve public speaking classes to learn more on organizing, presenting what you think and making you sound more convincing.

III. Pacing: In this step, you will learn how to establish similarities. You need to learn how to mirror your victim's body language, then see how effective you can control your tonal variations and other body languages. The gentle and manipulative technique is the best when persuading your employer or fellow employees to get them do something for you. In this case, you should NEVER be emotional since this is a professional setting.

IV. Be Charismatic: Once you are charismatic, you will have the tendency to get what you want. In this step, you need to learn how to smile and light up a room. You should as well have approachable body gestures so your targeted people feel willing to talk to you. You should be flexible such that you can hold up a discussion with anyone despite their age, body size, or profession. The following are other techniques you should apply to be charismatic:

• Making others feel special by maintaining eye contact when talking to them, asking them how they feel and what are their interests. Show them how much you care about knowing them even if you know you do not mean it.

• Love yourself and what you do by exuding your confidence. Have faith in yourself so others can take you seriously and fall into your persuasion intent.

• Be confident even if what you are saying is true or false. When speaking, be glib as this makes your target fall into your purpose easily.

V. Learn from Other Manipulators: Since you are still an amateur, you need to learn more from the masters. Look for your friends or family members who are persuasion masters and take notes. This helps in getting new insights on how to persuade and influence people even if it means you end up being a manipulation victim. If you are interested in the art of mind control, you might also find yourself manipulating one of the masters.

VI. Read People: You should also learn to read people as everyone has a different emotional and psychological composition and should, therefore, be persuaded for various purposes. Before you apply your latest manipulation skills, take time to learn your target by understanding what makes them tick, then evaluate which approach suits them. The following are the most proven factors you will come across when getting to know more about people:

• The majority are vulnerable to emotional responses. They are emotional themselves as they can cry while or after watching a movie; they love pets and are sympathetic. This means in order for you to persuade them, you will have to play with their emotions until they empathize and sympathize with you and give in to your intents.

• Others were raised in authoritarian backgrounds, hence have a guilt reflex. Since they are used to getting punished for every little wrong deed, they grow up feeling guilty about anything they do. As a manipulator, make them feel guilty for not fulfilling your demands, and within no time, they will grant your wishes.

• Other people are amenable to rational approaches. They are always logical-minded, tend to read the news every day, and they always ask for facts before deciding on anything. In this case, you will need to apply your calm mind-controlling powers to influence these people rather than using your emotions.

Apply Different Persuasion and Manipulation Techniques

I. Always Start with Unreasonable Requests in order to Get More Reasonable Ones: This step is a time-tested technique for persuasion. As a manipulator, you should always start with unreasonable demands, and then wait for the victim to deny you, then follow it up with a more approachable request. It will be hard for them to reject you for the second time, as the second request will sound more appealing as compared to the first request.

II. Ask for a Rare Request before Your Real Request: This is another way of getting what you want as it entails requesting a strange thing that throws your target off guard, making them unable to deny you. Then ask for the more usual type of request, and the victim will not be able to deny it since their mind has been trained to avoid these activities.

III. Stimulate Fear, Then Liberation: For successful persuasion, tell the person what they fear, and then relieve them of it, and with no doubt, they will be happy to grant your wish. It may sound mean, but you will get your results instantly.

IV. Make your Target Feel Guilty: Making your target feel guilty is another step for a successful manipulation. You need to start by picking someone susceptible to feeling guilty. This should be followed by making them feel like they are bad for not granting your requests, no matter how absurd it is. The following can be the unchallenging victims who will fall into your persuasion technique:

• Parents - Manipulate your parents by making them feel guilty. Mention to them how you feel your life is full of sufferings since childhood because they are not granting your wishes.

• Friends - Remind them of all the good deeds you have done for them or else tell them how they usually let you down.

• Significant partner - Conclude your quarrels by saying 'Okay- furthermore I expected this.' This will make them feel guilty about letting you down several times.

V. Bribe: In this step, blackmailing is not necessary to get your wishes granted. Bribe your victim with an unappealing present. You can as well offer something you would have done anyway. First, you should figure out what your targeted person wants or lacks at the moment, then try giving it to them. Secondly, do not make it sound like you are bribing, but portray yourself like someone who is willing to help your victim in return for something you want.

VI. Playing the Victim: Making yourself the victim is always a great manipulation technique. You should use this step sparingly and effectively to pierce your victim's heart and get what you want. You have to act like you are a wonderful person, philanthropic, and that you are always the victim of every evil on earth. Play dumb as it makes your victim believe you are honestly perplexed by why evil things always befall you. Saying 'It is okay- I'm used to this' makes your victim feel like someone who cannot help you wall you a number of times and this tactic will make you get what you want. Finally, always be pathetic.

'It is okay- I'm used to this'

VII. Apply Logic: This step works better for the rational-minded people. Logica; acts as the most excellent persuader, more so when you carry along with come-oriented whys and wherefores on how what you are after would benefit both of you. While presenting your case, do it calmly and rationally to avoid losing your control. If you want to manipulate a rational person, NEVER be emotional. In this step, act like your request is the only option you have, and your victim will judge the case your way.

VIII. Never Break Character: When your friend, family member, or co-worker tries to manipulate you, pretend to be more upset than them. Look more hurt and tell them you are even amazed and you did not believe they could ever think that about you. This will make the victim feel guilty and sorry for you.

Manipulating Anyone in your Life

Getting everything you want.

I. Your Friends: This is one of the final steps now that you have equipped yourself with the active manipulation steps. When it comes to your friends, it can be a bit harder since they know you well. But this does not mean you cannot manipulate them. You should never tell them you are trying to persuade them, as this might destroy your friendship. The following are the steps you should follow if it is in your friend's case:

• First, butter your friend(s) up. This is done by being friendly, doing small favors for them, and telling them how amazing they are to you, and this is done a week before you make a request for a straightforward indulgence. Do everything a friend is supposed to do without going overboard.

• Your friends should care for you, specifically when you are emotionally down, and this is a significant step to get what you want. This means your friends will do everything possible not to see you upset. Use the skills acquired in your acting class to make you look more emotional than you really are.

• Remind your friends of how amazing you have been to them and how you have sacrificed substantial space and time to save the friendship.

II. Your Significant Other: This is the simplest step. You have to turn your partner on and then ask what you want because, in this state, they can hardly deny you what you want. There are also some other ways to persuade your significant partner than this subtle route. Look sexy when making the request, and they will grant your wish based on how cute you look.

III. Your Boss: This step requires you to apply rational and logical approaches. You should NEVER show up at your employer's desk crying or manifesting your problems as the likely result for this is getting fired. You should instead be logical with your employer and back up your request with detailed explanations. Therefore, you should:

• Be a model employee a week before requesting a favor. This can be achieved through working late, keeping a smile always on your face, and even bringing pastries in the morning.

• Request the favor in an offhanded way. This entails requesting the support like it is no big deal. Rather than saying, 'I want to ask for something really important from you,' be casual as you request this or you might alert the employer about your intents.

• Manipulate the boss at the end of the day or during breaks. In the morning, employers are stressed about all the work they have to do for that day. Persuading your boss during these mentioned hours has the highest probabilities of being successful, as the boss will instead grant your wish rather than waste their time.

IV. Your Teacher: This step works better if you combine professionalism with emotions. You need to:

• Be a role model to the other students by arriving to class early enough, reading ahead of the teacher and being active in class work.

• Appreciate your teacher by telling them how great they are in a composed manner. Tell them how much you love the subject and how much you enjoy their way of teaching.

• Talk of how much you are suffering at home as this will make the teacher feel awkward and sorry for you.

• While talking about your private life, wait until the teacher gets uncomfortable, and for instance, offers to give you an extension to rewrite an assignment. Let your tone trail off and start crying. You can as well opt for walking on your way home as the teacher would not be able to withstand this and will end up granting your wish.

V. Your parents: You have the right to maximum parental care and persuading your parents is also one of the easiest steps. If the parents love and support you, be a model son or daughter a while before making your request. Help out around the house as much as you can, then when you start persuading:

• Make your request in a reasonable way. Do not sit down and have a big talk about your request. Make it hard for your parents to say no to your request.

• State your claim while doing other household chores, such as folding the laundry. This reminds them of how good you are.

• Tell your parents about your friends, how their parents have granted the wishes of your friends and why your parents should feel okay too and grant the request.

• Make them feel guilty by talking on how you will get every detail of either a concert you missed or blame them for ruining your life by causing you not to have significant experiences in your life.

Having learned the steps for successful mind control, and how easily you can influence your friends, parents, boss, teachers or significant other, you should also know how effortless it is to manipulate someone hangs on the impressions you have of them. You should always be deceptive, use your emotions, and persuade using the waterworks approach in a public place, then finally use bribes where necessary.

Chapter 9: Persuading and Influencing People Using Manipulation

Human being as a social being is in constant communication for many reasons, giving information, getting information, asking for help, making promises, telling your feelings and thoughts, or trying to learn someone else's feelings and thoughts, and so on. Communication is established within a certain structure and order. At this point, one should look at the definition of communication: Inter-human communication; It's the process of transferring information, emotions, thoughts, attitudes and beliefs and forms of behavior from one person to another through a relationship between the source and the recipient for change. As can be seen in daily life, in many situations where communication takes place, people either try to convince someone about the accuracy of the information they give, either to change their behavior or to convince them of something else because persuasion is an important and common reason for communication. The famous philosopher Aristotle defines communication as all the appropriate meanings of persuasion".

The concept of persuasion is defined in the dictionary as follows: Convincing, convincing; deceit; "Based on this definition, it will not be wrong to consider persuasion as a form of communication that is realized to achieve the desired aims." Indeed, when we look carefully, it can be seen that the difference between daily communication and persuasion is to achieve the desired goal. Not every communication phenomenon that is established in daily life is intended for persuasion, asking someone's memory only aims to learn about the person's condition and health. However, rather than persuading a person on a particular issue, it should be dealt with to uncover the desired change in the person who is exposed in the final analysis, which should be established with a certain systematic structure.

In the meantime, an important issue should be included here. It is also the effects of communication and how they occur. The effects of communication are:

1. Change in the recipient's level of knowledge

2. Changes in the attitude of the recipient

3. A change in the receiver's opens behavior.

In the second stage, the attitude change that came into the agenda is also realized in three ways:

1. Strengthening or strengthening the existing attitude

2. Change of existing attitude

3. New attitude formation

The effects of communication are often expected to occur sequentially and usually do. It is possible to see the effect of communication to a large extent in the change that may occur in open behavior. This is where the difference between daily communication and persuasion comes up. Persuasive communication is the expected and desired changes in attitude and open behavioral changes that will occur after the information is given. The attitude change that is expected to occur is determined by some attitude measurement techniques (Likert scale, etc.) developed in cases where open behavioral change can't be observed clearly or if it's not possible for different reasons, for example, an individual's Facebook, and so on. If it is desired to learn the attitude towards social media, a questionnaire consisting of expressions reflecting this attitude can be prepared. These statements; it allows people to share, enjoy the time, etc. can. It is possible to say that a Likert-type scale was used to measure the attitudes of the respondents to measure attitudes.

The concept and process of persuasion is a subject that has been studied intensively. In general, the biggest factors contributing to the success and failure of communication emerge as convincing communication and its proper structuring. With good understanding and knowledge of persuasive techniques; an educator, an advertiser, or a politician, in other words, it is possible to evaluate anyone whose purpose is to change the thoughts and actions of others. It should not be ignored that some essential variables exist in persuasion. Each of the variables in persuasion must be identifiable, distinguishable, and measurable. Scientists working in this field, these variables fall under two headings. These are called "dependent variables" and "independent variables. Arguments are made or occur with the communication process. We know what these variables will be, how they will be formed, and predict and produce their effects. Dependent variables, on the other hand, have to be done, and convincingly. We often hope to replace dependent variables with independent variables that we manage and control. Dependent and independent variables are called a convincing communication matrix.

The convincing communication matrix is a precise and complete data about all dependent and independent variables in human relationships throughout human life. Independent variables should be considered in many aspects and aspects of communication. However, dependent variables occur only when a person receives a persuasive message in terms of the information process. The main issue that needs to be emphasized about independent variables is the operation of the basic process of communication: "who, whom, what, through which channel and what kind of influences. The arguments that make up every convincing communication state appear in this case as "source, message, channel, receiver, and purpose. The dependent variables of the persuasive communication matrix are divided into six steps according to the characteristics of new behaviors, events, and phenomena in which the person is convinced. First, a convincing message must be presented. The second step is the participation of the target person in the communication, and this person needs to understand what is to be discussed. It's important that the recipient supports communication until the message is sent later and third. The fourth step is the understanding of the message, as well as the acceptance of the recipient or at least verbal adjustment. The fifth step is the most basic requirement. This step is the ability to accept until the effect can be measured. The sixth and last step or dependent variable is the ability of the target person to show the new behavior as open behavior. For example; depending on the main objective of the persuasion campaign, the purchase of a certain product, the selection of the candidate or leaving a harmful habit, etc. they are always concrete indicators of this last dependent variable. An analysis in the context of dependent and independent variables can help organize ideas about persuasion. The persuasion process is analyzed at all levels of communication.

These steps are as follows: Source of communication, form, content, and organization of communication, characteristics of the channel to which the message will be delivered, ability and characteristics of the intended recipient and intended behavior and attitude changes. Thus, under these five headings of communication, the efficiency of the persuasive communication process performed under the six steps of the dependent variables of persuasion is defined and evaluated. Examination of the persuasion process shows the importance of understanding and attention in a way. For example; when asked what kind of connection can be made between an intelligent buyer and persuasion, he will probably tell you that only a much smarter individual can convince that person. In other words, the more knowledgeable and intelligent person can only direct the person's point of view to another party. This point shows the variables of the connection between intelligence and persuasive communication. However, other points that should not be forgotten are the role and importance of attention and acceptance in the persuasion process.

Persuasion Techniques

The basis of persuasion is to direct the other person to the thought you desire and to make it normal in the basic belief and vision system. To simplify, it is to make the other person think the way you want. That's exactly what it means to convince. If the other person thinks the way you want, you can take the action that you want to take, that is, buying a product or consuming a product. Located below are techniques to persuade and convince some of the most effective techniques effectively. Persuasion techniques are not limited to these, but they are important for efficiency. You may encounter many other techniques of persuasion, such as rewarding, punishing, creating a positive or negative perception.

1. Creating Needs

One of the best methods of persuasion is to create a need or to reassure an old need. This question of need is related to self-protection and compatibility with basic emotions such as love. This technique is one of the biggest trumps of marketers in particular. They try to sell their products or services using this technique. The kind of approaches that express the purchase of a product to make one feel safe or loving is part of the need-building technique.

2. Touching Social Needs

The basis of the technique of touching social needs are factors such as being popular, having the prestige, or having the same status as others. The advertisements on television are the ideal examples. People who buy the products in these advertisements think that they will be like the person in the advertisement or they will be as prestigious. The main reason why persuasion techniques such as touching social needs are effective is related to television advertising. Many people watch television for at least 1-2 hours a day and encounter these advertisements.

3. Use of Meaningful and Positive Words

Sometimes it is necessary to use magic words to be convincing. These magic words are meaningful and positive words. Advertisers know these positive and meaningful words intimately. It is very important for them to be able to use them.

The words "New," "Renewed," "All Natural," "Most Effective" are the most appropriate examples of these magic words. Using these words, advertisers try to promote their products and thus make the advertisements more convincing for the liking of the products.

4. Use of Foot Technique

This technique is frequently used in the context of persuasion techniques. Processing way is quite simple. You make a person do something very small first because you think you can't refuse it. Once the other person has done so, you will try to get him to do more, provided that he is consistent within himself. First, you sell a product to a person at a very low price. Then you get him to buy a product at higher prices. In the first step, you attract him to yourself, so you convince him to buy it. In the second step, you convince yourself to buy products at a higher price. Their acceptance of a small thing will help you to fulfill the next big demand from you. After refusing the small request from the other party, you feel a duty to make a big request from the same person. This is usually the case in human relations. For example, you agree when your neighbor comes and asks you if you can keep an eye on the shop for a few hours. If your neighbor comes to ask you to look at the shop all day, you will feel responsible and probably accept it. This means that the technique of putting a foot on the door is successfully applied.

5. Use of Orientation from Big to Small

The tendency to ask from big to small is the exact opposite of the technique of putting a foot on the door. The salesperson makes an unrealistic request from the other person. Naturally, this demand doesn't correspond. However, the salesperson makes a request that is smaller than the same person. People feel responsible for such approaches, and they accept the offer. Since the request is small, by accepting it, people have the idea that they will help the salespeople and the technique of moving from big to small requests works.

6. Use of Reciprocity

Reciprocity is a term for mutual progress of a business. When a person does you a kindness, you feel the need to do him a favor. This is one example of reciprocity. For example, if someone bought you a gift on your birthday, you would try to pay back that gesture. This is more of a psychological approach because people don't forget the person who does something for them and tries to respond. For marketers, the situation is slightly different from human relations. Reciprocity takes place here in the form of a marketer offering you an interim extra discount" or "extra promotion... You are very close to buying the product introduced by the marketer you think offers a special offer.

7. Making Limits for Interviews

Setting a limit for negotiations is to provide an approach that will affect future copyrights. This is particularly effective when negotiating prices. For example, if you are trying to negotiate a price to sell a service, it might make more sense to start by opening the price from a higher number. Opening from a low number is not the right method because you have weakened your stretching share.

Even if the limitation for negotiations is not always useful, it's particularly useful in terms of price negotiation. Say the first number and get on with the bargaining advantage.

8. Limitation Technique

Restriction technique is one of the most powerful methods to influence human psychology. You can see this mostly in places selling products. For example, if a store has a discount on a particular product, it may limit it to 500 products. This limitation can be a true limitation or a part of the limitation technique. So you think that you will not find the product at that price again and you agree to buy that product at the specified price. The restriction technique is particularly useful in new products. As soon as a new product goes on sale, you can convince people to buy it for a limited time or by selling a limited quantity of products with extra promotions or discounts.

People who think that the product will not be sold again at a similar price may choose to buy the product you have chosen thanks to the success of your persuasion technique. Persuasion techniques are not limited to these. Different techniques can provide more successful results in various fields. However, most of the techniques that we may encounter in our daily lives consist of the methods here. If you want to be a marketer, if you are trying to sell a product or service, you need to have detailed information about these techniques if you want to make them available.

Difference between Persuasion and Manipulation

There are many similarities between Persuasion and Manipulation as the two words confuse non-English individuals: Natives too. There are many comparisons between the two concepts, and because of the overlap, people think these two can be used interchangeably. There are convincing good people, and there are good manipulators. Both try to make sense and encourage others to accept their views. However, although there are similarities in manipulation to making a cousin or persuasive sibling, there are differences to be emphasized.

Persuasion

Persuasion is a behavior from someone else directed in a specific direction. You've managed to convince when you try to explain a certain way of behavior logically and correctly, and others accept your opinion that they think is of mutual benefit. If you have good marks on your test and you asked your mother for an expensive gift, you are trying to convince her to buy you a gift. This persuasion is convincing because it sees the logic behind your request and buys gifts. The salesperson is persuaded to sell a product or service to customers as he tries to create the need for the product or service in the customer's mind.

Manipulation

Manipulation is the act of exploiting the instability of others and misleading them to accept your point of view. Manipulation is not mutually beneficial, only advantageous for the manipulator. At the subconscious level, people strive to control each other in an organization or a family. Instead of persuading them for their benefit, they try to manipulate them. Manipulation can also be for the good of the person, even as a child's mother says that instead of eating all of them from the cookie jar, they can get a cookie. This creates the possibility of illusion, and your child can easily accept for fear of losing the jar without a single cookie. You manipulated the child's behavior for his good. Manipulation can also be bad, and manipulation is bad because the manipulator aims to trick and benefit from it.

The distinction between persuasion and manipulation

• Manipulation, managing others to benefit flawlessly.

• Persuading a particular person to change his or her thinking logically and rationally by reasoning with himself or by presenting arguments

• Manipulators can achieve short-term success, but people know who is manipulated and who convinces them in the long run.

• Persuasion is the art of achieving what you want by creating changes in the behavior of others, but it is manipulation. However, the difference is your intention.

• A person with good communication skills but malicious intent is dangerous because he can be a good manipulator.

Popular Persuasion techniques:

Brainwashing

Influence in various ways to alienate man from his thought and worldview, to think and act in another direction. Man is a creature that thinks and is very wrong at the same time. Because no living thing is as open to human influences, both from its internal structure and from outside, it is not as influenced by human influences. Brainwashing is the exploitation of the human being's ability to be exposed to internal and external influences.

Brainwashing can be classified as being performed in a long and short term. Short-term brainwashing: This is a method of brainwashing using medical and psychological procedures. The essence of this method is the excitement of human beings by preparing tired, sleepless, drugged situations in which the said things are accepted without details, uncontrolled, it is to constantly influence it and put it into behavior that does what is desired without discussion. The founder of this method is the Russian scholar Pavlov. Pavlov concentrated his work on conditional reflexes.

"Reflex" is the body's reaction to a natural warning. The spontaneous withdrawal of the hand's approach to fire is an example. Conditional reflexes are reflexes that are dependent on habit and gained over time. Pavlov used dogs as test subjects. Many times he gave the dogs meat just after a ringtone. In later experiments, it was observed that the dogs drooled with the ringing sound even though no meat was given. Pavlov has given dogs various conditional reflexes. In 1924 there was a major water disaster in Leningrad. Pavlov's dogs flooded the building. The dogs stayed for days at elevated water levels up to their noses. After rescuing, it was seen that dogs lost their conditional reflexes. It was this event that led Pavlov to the brainwashing method. He concluded that events such as extreme fear, excitement, and fatigue erased acquired conditional reflexes. The next experimental tools were people who were victims of the communist regime. Such methods were developed so that the mental angels of a human being were disrupted, their memories and imaginations were erased, and with the logic of making, a robot personality with other emotions was created. The first condition for this was to bring about the mental collapse of dogs in humans. This is a state that has long been seen in humans and is called mental collapse. Pavlov developed new methods for creating a mental collapse. Four conditions were needed to ensure this.

1. Fatigue: The first thing to do to brainwash is to tire. For this reason, one is prevented from sleeping during long circuits. For example, by keeping strong light on the face, both fatigue and sleep are provided.

2. Astonishment: When the mental activities are weakened and solved by the effect of this big fatigue, the poor person is rained for hours of questioning. His mind is so confused that the connection between truth and lies is completely lost.

3. Permanent pain: Wounds open on your body that will last for a long time. It is connected to the clamp or chain, and its movement is prevented.

4. Continuous fear: The ways to create feelings of tension or fear is resorted to. As a result of these applications, the exhaustion of the human reaches its limit and image dissolves. The out of control of the mind has the following consequences: Person

is deprived of referral and effort. Memory clutter: Memories, interpretation, and reasoning skills; old habits are completely lost. The sequence of events has been forgotten. The nerves between the dream and the truth have become dark and blurry.

Melancholy: The mind wriggles in the grip of an unknown problem. One wants to commit suicide. Increased ability to be instilled: By taking advantage of this weak and defenseless state of man, they instill memory into a false form through suggestion. The new ideas they want to be believed are placed in the patient's tired mind as a form of suggestion.

The brainwashing process is now complete. Such a method of brainwashing has been used by the communist states, especially Russia and China. As a result of the brainwashing of the American soldiers who were captured by the Chinese in the Korean War; "We have seen the facts now. We were servants to the imperialists. The goal of communism is to achieve world peace. The Chinese couldn't apply brainwash to Turkish soldiers who were captured during the Korean War. Psychologists have shown the strength of faith in the Turkish soldier, their unshakable discipline and commitment to each other.

Long-term brainwashing: This method is carried out by propaganda. Propaganda: Persuasion, persuasion, deception, arousing suspicion, and intellectual and spiritual oppression activity. It is a sensitive and special method which is applied by having a positive or negative influence on the ideas, opinions, thoughts, and feelings of individuals and society.

Propaganda means; satellites, sports, and art activities, the press, television, radio, and books, they are the communist countries that give the most important to the brainwashing of people with propaganda. Russia has allocated 1/4 of its national income to propaganda. The aim of the propaganda is the human's ideas, feelings, that is, the spiritual. The brainwashed men are the prisoners of the enemy with a stronger chain of captivity than the first and medieval slaves. A wicked man who has been brainwashed against his nation and state can't understand that he is the slave of the enemy until the end of his life because of the values to show that what he did was bad. The measurement of value is only determined by having national and spiritual feelings and owning them. The person who loses these values acts according to the desires of the enemy. This is a slave, or rather a robot. The robot follows orders, for a normal person, the order was given to him as, suggestion, faith, and decides through the filtering of national values and reason. The degeneration of the human brain instead of arms, deflating intelligence, and ensuring the nation's morale and spirit in the direction of dispersion will be directed.

Chapter 10: Mind Control Techniques

Mind control

The term mind control has many definitions and interpretations, but the crucial thing to note is that it doesn't involve any sort of magic or supernatural ability; it just requires a rudimentary understanding of human emotions and behavior. Mind control can involve brainwashing a person, reeducating them, reforming their thoughts, using coercive techniques to persuade them of certain things, or brain-sweeping. There are many forms of mind control, and we could fill an entire book discussing all those forms, but for our purposes, we will look at the concept in general terms. Mind control means a person is trying to get others to feel, think, or behave in a certain way, or to react and make decisions following a certain pattern. It could vary from a girl trying to get her boyfriend to develop certain habits, to a cult leader trying to convince his followers that he is God.

Mind control is based on one thing: information. We have the thoughts and beliefs that we do because we learned them. When we are subjected to new information on a deliberate and consistent basis, it's possible to alter our beliefs, thoughts, or even memories. The brain is hardwired to survive, and towards that end, it's very good at learning information that is crucial for our survival. When you receive certain information consistently, your brain will start to believe it even if you know it's not true. For example, even if you are the most rational person out there, if you go online and watch 100 videos about a certain conspiracy theory, you will start to believe it to some extent. That explains why people who seem smart can end up getting indoctrinated into cults or even terrorist groups.

Mind control also works more effectively when one is dependent on the person who is trying to control his/her mind. Even in relationships that are involuntary, the victim can start buying the perpetrator's world view if they have been dependent on the perpetrator for a long time. That explains phenomena such as Stockholm syndrome (where people who are kidnapped or held hostage start being affectionate towards their captors and empathizing with their causes). The worst thing you can do is assume that you are too smart for mind control to work on you. Under the right circumstances, anyone can be persuaded to abandon their world view and adopt someone else's. Mind games are covert tricks that are deliberately crafted in order to manipulate someone. Think of them as "handcrafted" psychological manipulation techniques. While other techniques are applied broadly, mind games are created to target very specific people. They work best when the victim trusts the perpetrator, and the perpetrator understands the victim's personality and behavior. Most of the psychological manipulation techniques we have discussed thus far can be used when crafting mind games. A person who understands you will tell you certain things or behave in certain ways around you because they are deliberately trying to get you to react in a certain way. It almost always involves feigning certain emotions.

People who play mind games use innocent sounding communication to elicit calculated reactions from you. Psychologists refer to such mind games as "conscious one-upmanship," and they have observed that they occur in all areas of life. Mind games occur in office politics, personal relationships, and even in international diplomacy. At work, someone could try to make you feel like you are not up to the task so that they can steal an opportunity from you. In a marriage, your partner could make certain seemingly innocent slights against you so that you feel like you have something to prove, and you take a certain course of action as a result. In dating, there are "pickup artists" who use different kinds of tricks to get you to lower your guard and let them in. Mind control is not the whole of the vague information you hear in gossip, accompanied by conspiracy theories. It is the product of secret experiments with systematic studies dating back to World War II, perhaps older. Of course, the 20th-century totalitarian regimes, who wanted to robotize their subjects, also played a major role in this. Therefore, the first thing to note is that developing technology facilitates the mind-control efforts of the oppressors every year. Like Telegram scourge that happens today... But mind control; it is something that can be done without technology with the support of psychology and orator. The most striking example of this in history; this is the work carried out by Goebbels, the Minister of Propaganda of the Nazis. Goebbels succeeded in engraving his name in gold letters in this lane, which was the disgrace of humanity.

Mind control; It is the name given to all the unethical activities of some power centers to manage people in line with their goals, to shape their ideas and control their lifestyles. While technological opportunities can be utilized in mind control, human psychology, propaganda knowledge, and social engineering are essential.

Also, mind control; it is applied in a highly systematic, insidious way by people who have done as much research as required by a master or doctor. In other words, it is essential that people don't realize the engineering applied to them, so to be hypnotized. Therefore, it is challenging to recognize and resist. Also; every political and intellectual propaganda is not minded control. Mind control, as we mentioned above, is a different matter.

Effects of Mind Control on human

The effects of using mind control on human beings are seen in different ways. Some of them are as follows;

• "Memory loss and behavior disorders

• Change in direction, intensity and content of sound heard

• Speech deterioration by checking eyelids

• Severe heart palpitations

• Forcing accidents on the shoulders and arms during laborious work

• Jogging of the elbows and preventing work while doing something

• Pain and unnecessary movement of the legs, right and left swing and excessive stiffness

• Itching and blushing in hard-to-reach areas

• Contractions of large muscles in the back

• Checking hand gestures

• Reading thoughts or transmitting thoughts from outside

• Seeing moving imaginary images

• Keeping eyelids constantly open

• Continuous tinnitus

• Jaw and teeth shivering for no reason

Chapter 11: Manipulating Mass Opinion as a Public Speaker

Remember that earlier we talked about three different steps that have to come into play when it is time to work with influencing someone to do what we want. Whether we want them to finish a report for us, give us some extra tips, help us out with some work or with our kids so we can get a break, or even to sell them a product, we need to be able to use these three steps to help us get what we want from the target. First, you need to work on analyzing the other person. Depending on how long you plan to know this person and how much influence you plan to do, you will need to spend a bit of time doing an analysis to help you see success. Once the analysis is done and you have a good idea on what is going to work the best for your target, it is time to move on to manipulation or planting the seeds of what you want the target to do.

Once you have been able to work through some of the strategies that are presented in that chapter on your target, it is time to move on and learn a bit about how to work with persuasion to get what you really want. There are a number of steps that you are able to use in order to persuade your target. And you will find that a lot of these are easy, and maybe already done if you have gone through the two other steps and some of their techniques from earlier. When you are ready to start persuading someone to do what you want, make sure to follow some of the steps below to help you to get started! And overcome the trust issues that are there. One of the first things that we are going to work on is the idea of trust issues that could be there. It is possible that the person you choose for your target is someone you have just met. Or maybe you have known them for a long time and yet have had very little to do with them over the years. And now you want to come in and really get them persuaded to do something that they may not be that sure of on their own. There is bound to be some trust issues. It doesn't

144

matter how good you are with manipulation. And it doesn't matter how likable of a person you are in the beginning. What does matter is how much the other person trusts you. And you need to be willing to work on building up that trust, and learning how to overcome any trust issues if you really want to make sure that you get the best results here.

The good news is that there are a few steps that you are able to follow in order to really work on some of these trust issues. Once those are resolved, you will find that it is easier than ever to really work with persuasion and to get what you want from anyone. So, let's take a look at some of the different steps that you can take as a manipulator when it comes to trying to build up that trust that you want.

First, you need to make sure that you learn how to study the actions of other people. Often times we are going to because of hurt because we believe that there is some promise there that has never been held as true or taken care of. And sometimes that thing has nothing to do with you but something in the past that your target is now dealing with. Watching the actions of the other person, and learning what trust issues may be there, and how you can fix them, can help them to open up and value you way more than before. One of the best things that you are able to do to build up some trust is to ask a lot of questions. You are never going to know what the other person is mad about or what causes them to have some trust issues if you have no idea why they are mad about something or why they have the trust issues. You need to ask a bunch of questions to figure this out sometimes.

This can be done no matter what kind of relationship you have with the other person or not. If you find that you are a salesperson who is trying to sell a product questions can help you to figure out why the person hasn't purchased the product in the past, what issues they may have gone through with purchasing this item or another one that is similar in the past, and what you would be able to do to make it better. Maybe the customer is nervous about purchasing a car because the last few were sold to them by someone they trusted, but these vehicles ended up being duds and costing way too much. You can take that information and then work on how to make it a bit better so that they trust you. Even if you are trying to build up a long term relationship with the target than you would as a salesperson, you will be able to use some of the manipulations and some of these questions in order to help you to do this. The more questions you ask the person about their past, about some of their friends, about what they are looking for in the future, and more, the more likely it is that you are going to be able to figure out what may have broken their trust in the past, and what you are able to do to increase that trust in the future.

You can also work on gathering information as much as possible. Your friend may not trust someone, but that isn't a sign that someone shouldn't be trusted. And maybe this is what is happening with you and your target. They have a friend who doesn't trust you for one reason or another (they may have never met you in the past either), and so they just don't trust you either. Knowing this information, and then talking to the more logical part of that person, rather than the emotional side that is listening to the friend, it going to make a big difference in what you are able to do to build up some of that trust. Go slowly. There are going to be some relationships that you are able to jump right into, even when you are working with a target of manipulation. But then there are some of those that need to go a little bit slower. There are those who have been hurt in the past or those who are just naturally wary of others around them, and they will want to be careful with anyone they are interacting with.

If you decide to jump into the mix too quickly, then you are going to scare them away and they will want to have nothing to do with you. But when you are really able and willing to just take things slow and let people get to know you (or at least the story of you that you want them to know), you will find that it is much easier for you to really gain their trust. Trying to get the target to blindly trust you is just going to make them clam up even more and this makes the situation so much worse. Instead, talk to them slowly and give them some time to determine if they want to be in this kind of relationship, whether it is a romantic one, a friendship, a working relationship or something else or not. If you take it slowly, it also gives you more time to really work with some of the other techniques that we have talked about, which can make a world of difference in how much success you are going to see here.

It is so important for you to gain some level of trust with your target. Even though persuasion and manipulation don't seem to go hand in hand with trust, it is impossible to persuade your target to do anything that you want them to do. Building up some form of trust, whether it is a short term trust that you do in the spur of the moment as you meet them at work or one that you build up over time because of the long relationship that you are going to be in.

Know what your purpose is.

Before you ever try to persuade anyone to do what you want and before you use any of the other techniques that are found in this guidebook, you really need to make sure that you know what your purpose is. You don't want to do all of the work that is presented above, and then find out that it is not enough because you have no idea what your purpose is. This purpose is really going to drive all of the other things that you are going to focus on when it comes to working through this guidebook. We are going to focus on what we want to get the target to do. What actions are they able to take that will ensure we get what we want in the end?

If you are not able to answer that question, then it is hard to really have any idea of the steps that you need to take in order to make this happen. Think about what your purpose is here. Your main purpose is to get someone to do what you want so that you can reach your own goals. Sometimes this is going to be beneficial for both of you. This can be seen when the target comes in to purchase a car. You sell it which benefits them because they get a new vehicle, and you benefit because you made a sale and get to keep the money for your paycheck.

But with manipulation and persuasion, sometimes the result for the target is not going to be as positive. In fact, many dark manipulators are not going to care about how their actions are going to affect others. They just want to get the benefits that they need and feel that they deserve, and that is all that they are really going to care about at the time. This can be seen in manipulative relationships. The manipulator is going to woo someone into the relationship and will keep them there. The target is not going to receive much from this relationship, and often they are going to be harmed in the process and be emotionally, physically, and mentally drained by the end of it. But the manipulator doesn't care because they will feel like they got what they wanted for the length of the relationship. This is why we need to understand our purpose. If we don't understand why we are walking into the process of manipulation (to get what we want), it is possible that we will be turned around by emotions and not do what we set out to do. This could end with us not getting the sale, not getting the relationship, or not getting something else that we really wanted.

Be calm and confident.

As a manipulator, you really need to learn how to keep your emotions in check as much as possible. This is going to be one of those things that often seems easier said than done, but it is definitely something that you need to be able to focus on as much as possible.

Think of it this way, if you say someone comes over to you who seemed to be a bit agitated, or they were snickering with an evil grin on their face how likely is it that you would give them the time of day? It is likely that you would turn away and want to have nothing to do with them at all because you would feel like something was up.

And this is exactly the same way that the target is going to feel if you are not careful about how you react to situations around them. You need to be willing to stand up for yourself, be calm, and be confident, in order to ensure that the target feels comfortable with you and to ensure that they are not going to feel like something is up before you even get a chance to speak with them.

First, we need to take a look at the steps to remaining calm around the target. You do not want to come up to them sweating, heavily breathing, bouncing around, and acting like you are nervous. Sure, it's +very possible that you do feel these things. But on the outside, it is going to look really suspicious and it is going to be really hard for you to build up any of that trust or that connection that you need with the other person at all. If you are able to come up to your target with a lot of confidence, and you are able to show them that you have no fear, and you are sure in yourself, in your message, and in what you have to say to them, then this issue is gone. Now, it is normal for you to feel a little bit antsy and anxious when you are first starting out. That is the beauty of practice when it comes to working with persuasion. Over time you will get a lot better. If you still find that the nerves are bothering you and you are not able to get them under control, you have a few steps at your disposal as well.

Before approaching the target, take a few slow and cleansing breaths in and out to let it all go. Count down or up from ten, and see if that is able to help clear your head, get the shaking to go down, and will help you to stay as calm and collected as possible. The next thing that we need to concentrate on is the idea of adding some confidence to your stance and to your life. Confidence is hard to do, but it is something that you are able to fake a bit in order to convince someone else that you possess a lot of confidence, even if it is not really there for you. If you are worried about how to do this, then some of the steps to make you appear more confident to everyone around you, even though you may be sweating bullets and feel like there is no confidence around you at all, includes:

1. Avoid your pockets: Those hands need to stay out of the pockets. Put them almost anywhere else, but do not let them get lodged into your pockets and out of site.

2. Do not fidget: When you are nervous it is easy to spend some of your time fidgeting and not able to sit still. This is a clear sign that you are tense, hiding something or worried. When you become more conscious about the fidgeting that you are doing, you will find that it is easier to make it stop, and confidence is going to follow.

3. Keep the eyes forward: Nervous people are going to glance all over the place except at the person they are talking to. We have already talked a bit about why this is a bad thing and the importance of eye contact, so make sure that your eyes are on the target, and not glancing all around the room in a nervous manner.

4. Stand up straight: Not only does slouching make you look bad and like you are unorganized, but it is also going to look bad when it comes to how much confidence you have in yourself. Make

sure that when you meet with anyone, but especially with your target, you stand up nice and straight with your back up and your shoulders back. No matter how nervous you are, this kind of stance is going to really make a difference in how much confidence people have in you.

5. Take steps that are wider: Don't go crazy with this one. If you are short, your steps are not supposed to reach so far that you fall over or anything. But if you are taking steps that are quick and short, then it may feel like you are sneaking, creeping, or scurrying, and these are not words that are used when it comes to someone who is confident. Do a nice stance while you walk (based on your own height), and see what a difference it makes in the confidence you have.

6. Firm handshake: We have all had that one handshake that never seems like it is completed. You have to pretty much do all of the work of holding onto the hand, much less making sure the handshake gets done. Don't be like this. Use a

firm handshake that is going to impress all of those around you.

7. Proper grooming: You have to take care of yourself when it comes to showing others that you are really confident in yourself. Keep your hair nice and kept up on a regular basis, wear clothes that are meant to impress, brush your teeth, take a bath on a regular basis, and make sure that you wear some perfume or cologne that is a nice scent, but not too overpowering.

8. Smile There is nothing better to helping out with your confidence and making you appear better to others than smiling on a regular basis. When you are confident, you really have no reason to worry about anything. Try this little experiment for a moment. The next time that you are walking down the street or the hall at work, give someone a smile. Chances are pretty high that this person is going to smile back at you. This is because you show confidence and it helps to rub off on them as well. You can do this with your

target as well when you are working on that confidence.

9. Don't have your arms crossed when you are socializing: When you cross your arms, it is showing that you are trying to protect something. This is an action that we are going to do when we are on guard, nervous, or cold. And none of these things are going to inspire a lot of confidence, are they? It is important to do something else with your hands. Put them casually by the side. Or, if this seems a bit off, you can consider using hand gestures to help get your point across while still having something to do with your hands.

10. Use contact when you want to show some appreciation: A pat on the back is something that is considered a lost art in our society. But it can not only sow some of your own confidence, but it is going to be a great way to feel closer and more connected to the target when you need. Be careful with this and only use it with those who are going to be comfortable with your actions.

As you can see, there are a number of things that you are able to do in order to make sure that your target is going to see you as calm and confident all of the time. You will be amazed at how the projection of these two character traits are going to get people to jump at the chance to do what you want, and they are easy things that you can learn without a ton of practice or hard work along the way.

Manipulate the body language that you are using.

The next thing on the list that you are able to work with is manipulating your own body language. Many people think that this is just something we can't do at all. We assume that because we often don't think about our body language, there is no way that we are able to manipulate it to do what we want it to. While it is true that a lot of body language can happen on its own, without us even thinking about it, this doesn't mean that we can't put some control with it. It is going to take some work, but it can be done.

First, we need to take a look at the different things that you are able to do to start adding in some manipulation to your body language. Start with the face. For the most part, you will want to make sure that you have a smile around your target. This is going to make them feel more comfortable around you, and can really open up the lines of communication that you both have. However, a true smile and a fake smile are completely different. The fake smile only pulls up the corners of the mouth, and many of us are able to spot this kind of smile and we won't form the connection with it like other options. A real smile is going to involve the whole face, from the mouth to the eyes and everywhere in between. Go in front of a mirror and see if you can tell the difference. Put on your fake smile, the one that you use when you want to be polite or you are trying to smile to someone you meet in the hallway. Now think of something that makes you really happy, something that can always get you to smile, and put that on your face. Notice a difference? Your goal is to get the second one to show up each time that you talk to your target.

Next, we need to work with the eyes. You are not going to keep the attention of your target if you are constantly looking away or trying to look at your watch or something else. This gives off the appearance that you are either trying to hide something from them or that you would rather be somewhere else. And neither of these are going to give a great opinion of you to the other person. You also don't want to stare the other person down because this is going to greatly intimidate them, and that isn't going to help you out at all either. Rather than doing this, your goal is to use some natural and easy eye contact to ensure that there is a level of comfort there. You will notice that when you are able to maintain eye contact, without staring the other person down like you want to scare them, that it is much easier to get them to feel comfortable around you, and for you to make that connection that you want. Next is the hand gestures. You want to make sure that there are some being used in all of this. Keeping your arms stiff and right next to you is not going to work. But moving the arms around and making sure that they are used to talk about your point and in the right amount, can make a world of difference. Try to find a happy medium between arms crossed and arms that are flailing all over the place and about to hit someone else.

Your stance is important as well. You need to make sure that you have a good, straight posture the whole time. Slouching is not going to put you in the best light with the other person, and just doesn't give you the confidence that is needed to do well and leave a good first impression. While we are at it, work to make sure that your body is pointing in the right direction. To show the target that you are really interested in what they are saying and where this conversation is going, you want to make sure that your feet and body are turned towards them, and that you lean in a little bit to them as well. These are just a few of the things that you are able to do in order to manipulate your own body language when you are around the target. Adding these in can be as easy as you make it but the point is to make sure that every part of your body shows that you are interested in the target and that you want to make a connection. If any part of your body language goes against this, then it is going to mess with the message and can make the target feel like you are trying to hide something from them along the way as well.

Practice guilt trips.

When it comes to manipulation, there is nothing that is used as often as the guilt trip. This is going to ensure that the manipulator is able to get what they want. And they are so successful with it because they can use the emotions of their target against them in the process. The manipulator, even when they are the ones in the wrong, are going to be able to use this kind of resource in order to get the target to acknowledge the fact that they (manipulator) did a lot of things wrong, or that they are the ones to blame. This takes any of the responsibility from the manipulator and places it all, unfairly, on the target.

So, how do we use the idea of a guilt trip to get what we want? First, you need to start bringing up the conversation of what went wrong and talk about how this person has done other similar things in the past. There is usually going to be some story that goes on with it and makes them feel bad. They may say, "You never have time for me anymore. Remember last week I needed help with something and you didn't have time. And now today I need help and you are too busy again."

This brings up the idea that the target is never there for the manipulator when the manipulator needs them. Never mind the fact that the target was maybe stuck in traffic and couldn't get home last week or they are horribly sick this week and that is why they can't help. It is all about what the manipulator wants and needs, and they are going to use that guilt trip to get it. In this step, the manipulator is going to make the situation seem so much worse than it is. They may sigh and act disappointed by the fact that this is now a type of behavior pattern that they expect, and that they don't really deserve to be treated this way all of the time either. It is most effective when the manipulator is able to surface matters that are comparable to whatever they want their target to admit to doing wrong, even so it can really be used to bring up anything that upsets you.

This whole process is going to really play on the feelings that the target has for the manipulator. The manipulator is going to take the time to let the target know that they now query how they do feel about them (manipulator). In other circumstances, this may be true, but in reality, the manipulator is just doing this in order to prey on the target and make them feel bad. The point here is to get the target to feel so bad that they want to prove how they care about you (the target) and they want to make it better. The manipulator may also spend some time reminding the target of all the sweet good things they have been doing for the (the target) in the past. They are going to put the supposedly bad actions of the target in light of all the good things that they have been able to do for the target over time. The grander the gesture that the manipulator is able to pull out, the better this is going to be. And often the action doesn't have to relate with the topic at hand, just as long as the manipulator comes out looking like they are on top.

Now, you have to remember that in many cases, the target is going to try and point the finger back at you. This is especially true if the situation is the fault of the manipulator, rather than of the target. But your job is to put as much, if not all, of the guilt on the other person, so you need to deflect any other efforts if any to actually make or turn the whole situation into something that is your fault. Even if you have done something in this situation that is wrong, you should not accept it at all. If anything, it is much better if you are able to turn it all around reflecting what your target did.

For example, maybe you really need your partner to apologize because they were texting someone else. They may try to turn this around and ask why you went through their phone in the first place. Instead of admitting that what you did was something wrong, you would turn the conversation back on them and tell the them "Well, it actually seems I had enough reason to suspect that something was not right, didn't I?

And finally, make sure that you are able to bring up the feelings or if you like emotions that bring about the guilt trip as much as possible. If the target is really fighting against this and they are resisting all of your attempts of this guilt trip, then it is time to resort to some of the drama. This is where stomping around, yelling, crying, and any other big emotion is going to come in. Sometimes this works because the other person is going to say anything and everything you want in order to get you to feel a bit better. Remember, the point of working with the guilt trip is to get the other person to take the blame and the responsibility of something that went wrong. It doesn't matter in manipulation if they are the ones to blame or not. Once they accept this blame, the manipulator has the control. The target is going to want to do something in order to get that trust back or to release the blame, and they will turn to the manipulator to figure out how to make this happen.

Play the victim.

The next thing that you can work on is playing the victim to your target. This kind of tactic is always going to see you as the one who is downtrodden, the one who is not getting the attention that they deserve, and who is being treated unfairly all of the time. This is a tactic that is going to work the best on those who like to feel and take care of things based on their emotions. This is because their aim is to aid the manipulator, not realizing that most of the stories they are hearing from the manipulator are made up and not really true. When it comes to playing the victim, no one is going to be better at it then the manipulator. They know how to play the victim better than anyone else around them. They can make you feel guilty about almost anything that they want, without batting an eye about it either.

It always seems like the world is going down hard on the manipulator when they play the victim.

Someone was unfair to them at work. The neighbor's dog was barking too much (Even though they brought the dog in at 9), and they were not able to sleep. They thought you were mad at them and this caused them a lot of anxiety. They found out that they were passed over for a promotion and it isn't fair, even though they never get their work done on time and have only been at the business a few months. It seems like the manipulator is able to complain about everything and anything under the sun. It is all out to get them, from other people, the word, and every situation that they encounter. It doesn't matter that they have done nothing to make the situation better and that often they have purposely tried to make it worse to guilt trip the target. And it doesn't matter if the target has had a bad day as well for some legitimate reason. No one has had it worse ever than the manipulator, and the target is expected to feel sad and guilty about that fact.

This is a technique that is going to play on the emotions of the target. The hope here is that the target, even if they had a bad day or aren't feeling the best either, will feel bad or sorry for the manipulator and what that person is going through. They will be there to provide some level of comfort, and maybe they will even try to make things easier in another way. They may get the manipulator that promotion, wait on them hand and foot at home, and to other things in the hopes of making things a little bit better for the manipulator. Of course, things are never going to get better. The world is always going to be out to get the manipulator in some manner or another. This is just how things work in this kind of relationship. If the manipulator started to say that things were getting better, then they would not get the love and attention that they wanted from the target, and they would lose that amount of control. And if you find that you are able to get the target to do what you want after these sessions of playing the victim, know that you have the control over them that you want.

Use the logic that you have to appeal to rational people.

If you are working with a target who is really into the logic, and really into the idea of needing to know the facts and the figures before making the decision, then this is what you will need to focus on. It is not going to do you much good to bring out the emotions with this kind of target. It isn't that this kind of person isn't going to respond to emotions or that they don't have any emotions. But they are going to form a bigger connection with the facts and figures instead, and being able to point them in this direction is going to make a world of difference. When you want to be able to manipulate this kind of person, you want to make sure that you are able to bring in a lot of facts and figures to the mix. Show them, with studies, math numbers, and more, why this method is going to be the best one for them to work with. Let them see how it is going to benefit them by really saving money, how it is going to be good for so many reasons, and so on.

The more logic that you are able to add into the mix, the better this is going to work. You do not want to worry about the emotions or anything like that. If you are able to write up a report with all of the facts and figures, then this could serve you well. Don't worry if you can't, but it's the idea that you need to really think through the actions and the argument so that you can appeal to this kind of person as much as possible.

Inspire fear and then provide some relief to the person.

Fear can be a powerful motivator to get someone to do what you want. But remember that it needs to be done with a certain amount of delicacy. You can't go through this process and start causing fear right after you have met the person. If you haven't done your analysis or worked with some of the manipulation techniques from the last section, then this is going to end really badly. The other person may become fearful of you and never come around you again, or they may decide that you are just going to use these tactics against you and walk away from the relationship.

You have to form some kind of connection with the target first. This will help to keep them around, to ensure that they stay with you, even when the fear is there. It takes some time, but it can make the target feel like they need to act and behave in a certain way in order to avoid the anger and the fear from you and to really keep things smooth.

Adding in the fear is something that is going to scare the target quite a bit. They don't want to be fearful of anything. They don't want to feel like something is wrong or like they are walking on eggshells. And if they have a good connection with their manipulator to start with, they are going to do whatever they can to avoid this feeling and get things back on track.

If you are able to inspire this fear in your target, and then offer them a path they can take to make things better, to make sure that you are happy (and in their minds, they are happy too), then the target is going to do what you want. They will learn what inspires the fear, and what inspires the relief, and they will start toeing the line and doing what they are told in the process.

As you can see, there are a lot of different methods that can be used when it comes to adding persuasion into your influence of other people. It takes some practice and it is not always as easy as it seems. But you will find that if you do all three of these sections together, and you take your time with them rather than rushing to the manipulation, they are going to start falling naturally into place as well.

Chapter 12: Dealing with Manipulation and Manipulating People

It is one thing to understand manipulation, and how it works and can wreak havoc on your life. Understanding all the different tricks and tactics that a manipulator can use against you. May make it seem like it is impossible to defend yourself against manipulation. But the truth is that by understanding in excellent detail how manipulators can use a wide array of tactics against you. You use their weapons against them, something they are not expecting. To understand a potential enemy and the tactics they might use is to beat them at their own game. Too often manipulators enter our lives because we find their companionship pleasing, we let them fill a need that they create. This need can come from many places, for some a broken home, for others a simple need for action. To not know yourself is the greatest asset a manipulator can use against you. They act like parasites burrowing their way into your life and sucking you dry, getting all that they can resource-wise and then leaving you.

The good news is that you can avoid having this happen to you if you don't let it. Too often we let people dictate how they can treat us by our actions. If we let someone convince us that we are weak and need them to succeed than is it their fault for us getting sucked into their web. Or is it perhaps our fault for convincing ourselves that this "relationship" is good for us. The truth of the matter is that manipulators like to prey on people who have been hurt before. Their charm, and glib cons us into thinking that they will help us with whatever issue we are dealing with. It may sound cold or blunt but by keeping your guard and check and not letting yourself get too close to someone upon meeting them you can quickly avert any potential mishaps or crisis that may come forward within that relationship.

I would also like you to consider that for some individuals their manipulation is pathologic, meaning that there is some underlying mental illness that is causing them to behave this way. These types of people are the most dangerous for the simple fact that they do not realize that they are doing anything wrong, Think of your sociopaths or bipolar. For others their tendencies for manipulation can be linked to a faulty maturation process, they think that it will always be their way or the highway. In the end, the motivations remain the same for all manipulators when boiled down and simplified, they want what they want, and they are going to get it by whatever means it takes.

Being confident is your first step in averting a manipulative attack, depending on the type of manipulation used you are going to want to be confident in different areas. The manipulation that a salesperson might use varies greatly than the type of manipulation a jaded lover would use on you, so knowing how to respond to each is paramount. For example, if you know a car is cheaper than someone is saying is be firm in your argument and do not let up ground. The same can be said if you suspect your partner of lying in a romantic relationship. By showing dominance in an encounter you say to the manipulator that you are not someone who will fall for their bait, you will not be their plaything. Moving on from just simply being confident and knowing your situation, there is de-escalation. Many manipulators when confronted about their behavior like to make the stakes of a situation seem higher than they are. With their end goal being that you will back off and drop the conflict out of fear.

Their goal is to scare you into submission, through whatever means required. Some will threaten suicide, some will threaten you directly, in the hopes you will back down. The trick here is to call their bluff and remain firm in your conviction that you know they are just trying to manipulate you.

Do not buy into their bluffs as once a manipulator realizes they can get away with something once they will do it again and again. As you set a precedent for them that manipulative behavior is okay. Calling a manipulators bluff in a high-tension scenario like this, in the beginning, may lead to them getting irater and more irrational. But if you are firm and stand your ground, they will quickly come to terms with the fact that they will not win here. The other component of de-escalation is not losing control of your own emotions, manipulators are very good at learning what buttons to press to set you off. Understand this when interacting with them, because if you just buy-in and get as angry and irrational as them then you are stooping to their level and letting them get what they want from you, which is usually attention. There are some simple calming techniques you can use when you feel your emotions brewing up. Take a slow deep breath and count to five in your head, you can also try peaceful imaging. Imagine yourself on a calm beach or somewhere pleasant to draw your mind away from the situation with the manipulator. Presenting yourself as calm shows a potential manipulator that you won't stoop to their level and are willing to not compromise your integrity. De-escalation tricks are pointless if you do not take active steps to change things from there, this can be as simple as trying to set firm boundaries. The way you do this is that you let someone know what your limits are what you won't put up with, for example, if someone lies to you and you catch them you are firm and consistent with the consequences of it. If establishing boundaries and trying to de-escalate the situation don't work, then it may perhaps be in your best interest to reduce the amount of contact you have with the manipulator.

Going low or no contact with a manipulator guarantees you that they cannot harm you. The problem with doing this is remaining firm in your conviction, it is very easy to tell someone that you are going to stop contacting them but doing it is much more challenging.

Once a manipulator feels you are pulling away, they will ramp up their scheming in the hopes they can entice you into staying with them. Simply put leave them to block their number and possible leave any friends you both shares. Manipulators love to use other people to do their bidding. This allows them to act through proxies and avoid arousing suspicion that they are the ones responsible for certain behaviors. You may find that the more challenging part of reducing contact with someone who is a manipulator is the obstacles you set yourself. Manipulators like to make you second guess yourself and doubt your instinct in the hopes that you will follow through with their intentions. This is why knowing certainly how you want to act is important. Take time to do your diligence before making any major decision pull back for a little bit and analyze all the facts at your disposal.

By taking a calm and measured approach to your decisions and actions you present an image of someone who is not weak. This more than anything will prevent you from becoming a victim of manipulators attacks. Because it represents the image that you are in control of their emotions and as a result can't have your own emotions used against you, as manipulators commonly try to get you to do. In closing know that you have a basic understanding of some of the methods manipulators use and how to defend yourself against them. You are now better able to understand where manipulation truly comes from and what drives people to use someone's own emotions against them. As a result of knowing how their weapons work you can utilize them in tricky situations in life, where they may prove incredibly useful. Because manipulation is so common in today's fast-paced world it is imperative for you to understand it if you want to get ahead. That is why I would like to discuss how psychological disorders play in manipulative behavior. Since these personality disorders present themselves as continues displays of abhorrent behavior it is easy to recognize them when you know the signs. The three most common disorders that make people prone to manipulative behavior are Antisocial Personality Disorder (APD), Narcissistic Personality Disorder (NPD), and Borderline Personality Disorder

(BPD). Understanding the pathologies and behaviors characterized by these kinds of psychological disorders allows you to quickly weed out people who could potentially be manipulators. While it may seem cruel to avoid someone because they have a "disorder" when it comes to your wellbeing and security you can never be too careful.

To begin the conversation on disorders that make one manipulative I would like to start with the lesser-known Borderline Personality Disorder or BPD. BPD as a disorder is characterized by an intense pattern of instability in both interpersonal relationships and sense of self, this instability is accompanied by an extreme of abandonment, when combined with the general impulsiveness and mood swings BPD brings make for a perfect storm of destructive behavior. Since individuals with BPD have such an intense fear of abandonment they may lie and manipulate to keep you closer to them while at the same time getting angry at you for spending so much time with them. This splitting between their desires and fears is where the term borderline comes from, their emotions are always bordering on the edge. Ever so close to teetering off and having a nuclear meltdown but still so far away. Often people with borderline personality disorder present their symptoms in a chaotic or disorganized fashion, which reflects the fact that they are unsure of who they are themselves. It is not known what causes an individual to develop a borderline personality disorder, but it is theorized that growing up in an abusive home or experiencing severe trauma at a young age makes someone more likely to develop it. An individual with Borderline personality disorder may be able to lure you in with how they may appear to make themselves vulnerable.

They are prone to sharing intimate details with their life very early on in a relationship in the hope of establishing trust and moving the relationship along quickly.

This where the instability in relationships comes to play, a person with a borderline personality disorder will want to move a romance or relationship much quicker than it should be. Their reasoning for this is their fear of being abandoned, this fear drives their whole being to such an extent that they will burn all their bridges in the ill-guided hope of keeping you. One of the final characterizations of BPD is a repeated pattern of intense tantrums and meltdowns when people leave them, for lack of a better word when this fear of abandonment ends up coming true due to self-sabotage borderlines have a bad tendency to self-destruct and burn down everything in their path.

Your best defense against a borderline is leaving before you are too involved. If someone wants to move a relationship quickly in a direction you don't feel comfortable with then it is in your best interest to leave while you can and when you have not invested much emotion. Moving on from one of the least known disorders, I would like to discuss a disorder we have all heard of Narcissistic Personality Disorder or NPD.

NPD is characterized by extreme self-centeredness and an inability to comprehend and understand the consequences of their actions. Because of this inability to understand consequence narcissists tend to repeat the same self-destructive behavior over and over again. We have all heard this term used to describe someone. Few of us actually understand what narcissism truly looks like. We are quick to label any behavior we don't like as narcissism when in reality it is subtler than that. Narcissists are not the overt self-centered people the media likes to portray them as. A narcissist likes to utilize subtle tactics to get you to come in line with their way of thinking, as opposed to overt manipulation. By getting you to question your judgment they can replace your ideas with theirs. One of the main behaviors all narcissists follow is the inability to take responsibility for their actions.

They will pin the blame for their actions on others instead of realizing that they are the reason misfortune keeps befalling them. As a result of this inability to learn from past mistakes, the narcissist will often repeat the same behavior over and over again to try and meet the same goal. This is what makes them so dangerous, they are willing to go to extreme measures to get their goals. The largest danger from narcissists comes from what is called a narcissistic meltdown. When a narcissist feels cornered like an animal, they will meltdown and destroy everything in their path even if it means damaging themselves. This can take many different forms, for some narcissists, this means something as extreme as suicide or even murder. For others, they may trash a lover's house when asked to leave the relationship. In short, when a narcissist realizes their game is up, they tend to blow a lot of fuses in their heads.

It is hard to postulate what motivates a narcissist as to behave this way current psychological research, points to a poor sense of self. But the truth is it does not matter why they do something that matters is your ability to avoid it. Narcissistic manipulation mainly takes the form of what is called gaslighting. Which in simple terms is the act of getting you to question your judgment of a situation and get you to think that you're the one with the issues and not them? By getting you to question your own beliefs regarding their behavior a manipulator is then able to live rent-free in your head! This is extremely dangerous behavior because it allows for self-doubt to be reinforced and allows for the manipulator to instill dangerous thoughts and ideas into someone's head.

The main thing to look out for in someone who behaves like this is how they were in past relationships if you see a pattern of them avoiding any responsibility for their actions then run away immediately. Manipulators can accomplish gaslighting through a variety of ways the main method in which they try to manipulate you is by breaking you down over time, slowly wearing away at you with the same line of garbage over and over again till you are forced to believe it. Once a narcissist has convinced you of their positioning it is very difficult to get a clear view, they obfuscate the truth and lie at every chance they have to try and get you on their side. They'll make you feel guilty for not going along with their behavior

The fact that this happens over a slow time is what makes it so damaging, it becomes difficult for you to realize that the behavior you are being presented with isn't normal, and usually by the time you have realized it is already too late. Narcissists are great at luring you back into their grips through very clever manipulation tricks, by subtly getting you to doubt yourself they slowly hook their tendrils into every aspect of your life until you feel powerless without them. The trick to getting past this kind of manipulation is just biting the bullet and running away. This can be hard to do because narcissists are very charming and good at convincing you, they will change. But the truth is a narcissist is never going to change their manipulative behavior is only going to get worse and continue. One of the narcissist's other dangerous weapons is to break down self-esteem in others. For instance, imagine you're an architecture and you are working on a new model for a house. Your manager gives you the rough blueprint, which you noticed there are a few areas that could use some improvements. You begin sketching your blueprint version and proceed to make a cardboard model of what they envisioned. A week later, your manager comes to see your progress, to which her face shows frustration. Raising her voice, she points out the different designs from hers, comments on how the rooms look too small and talk about how the deadline is in two weeks. Situations like these, where you are bombarded with criticism, figure out if what they're saying is constructive or destructive. Whichever one you decide it is, you want the person to get all their criticism out before trying to amend what you have done, since they will most likely ignore you while in such a state. Quietly take their words and wait until they're finished.

Afterward, explain whatever changes you made and your reasons for doing such a thing.

It is always good to know before being confronted if the change was worth it or not, so make sure to evaluate all your decisions. In any case, ask her to clarify her opinion. There is a good chance she will explain what she meant. However, if she were to dismiss your explanations and continue criticizing, at that point you can safely take her words for a grain of salt. And realize that the comments may not be reflective of what is truly going on in the situation. And instead, consider that what she is saying may simply be an attempt to manipulate you and get you to do something she wants.

Accepting that you are in a destructive relationship with a narcissist. Can be a difficult thing to do but once you start to look at all the signs together it ends up making sense. Someone who is going out of their way and lies and get you to believe things only through their worldview is not someone you want to be with. That is perhaps the saddest part of the manipulation. It doesn't tend to change and happens to only get worse as time moves on. Taking this examination of a relationship to the heart is required evil in the world we live in today. Perhaps arguably the most common form of manipulation in today's fast-paced society is the manipulation that salespeople will try and use on us. Most sales tactics play on simple human emotions such as need or desire, and very specific fears like a fear of missing out or not belonging. Advertisements target us so subtly that we do not realize we are being taken for a ride until we make a purchase that we do not need. By using fancy colors and enticing cinematic, advertisements can play on very primal parts of our brain and get us to do what they want.

Look at the newest advertisements for the iPhone, and how they show people who happy while using their fancy brand-new iPhone. Are they truly happy because of their new iPhone or is it perhaps the situations they are shown in?

The first step any successful advertisement has to take in getting you to buy its product is to convince you that you need it. How can they sell you something if you don't need it? Simple, they do so by creating these huge social media marketing campaigns in which they show thousands of people lining up to buy the newest and greatest fancy phone. They can convince you that if you want to be one of the cool kids that you should also buy into needing something you don't need at all, such as the new iPhone.

This manipulation works by playing on a psychological concept called "the fear of missing out". Your fear of not keeping up with the curve will entice you to buy the product even if it sets you back financially and even if you don't need it. You may have noticed how in lots of stores the kid's toys are all colorfully lit and have cool and interesting cut-outs designed to catch the attention of your little tyke. These bright colors and exciting stimuli fire up the reward centers of our brains and get us primed to make a purchase.

The other trick salespeople will try and utilize is the "fake sale".

You are probably wondering what I mean when I say fake sales, well simply put say an item has a sticker on it that says was 15 dollars now ten dollars, you will assume that is on sale and if you buy it now, you're getting a good deal. Well, the truth is much different than the reality you assume it to be the item is always marked as "on-sale". By marking playing on this fear of missing out, salespeople manipulate you on a very primal and basic level, as such it can be hard to avoid and defend against it.

Your best defense is knowing how much something is worth before you purchase it. Do your diligence and research prices of the item in question, shop around at different outlets to get an idea of what it is truly worth. This is especially important when purchasing a car, as the stereotypes about used car salespeople exist for a reason. They will tell you whatever you want to hear about a vehicle. Their main trick is trying to quickly get a read on you and discern your likes and dislikes once they do this, they can lure you into thinking they're your friend. And a friend will always give you the best deal, right? This is not always the case the people who are in this industry are in it because of the good people-pleasers they know what to say to people and how to get what they want from them. You can utilize some of these tricks in your own life, the main thing to remember when interacting with someone, is to make them feel validated and special. By doing this you get their trust, and from there, you can go far. Feeding into the fact that car sales are mostly a trick. There is also real estate where a realtor will try and convince you that something, you're going to invest in will only grow in value and you are missing out by not purchasing it.

They will try to woo you with stories about how great the local farmers market is and how their produce is so fresh, or how the schools in the area are so highly rated, but the truth is these things are usually just embellishments or flat out lies. One thing you may have noticed when looking at a potential house to buy is how the realtor may have baked cookies or how there will be premade candies or cakes. This is to get you to believe that the house is lived in and this also plays on strong mnemonic cues, humans associate smells strongly with emotion, as a result, we are quick to dismiss logic, and we will just go with our heart and ignore the facts.

All manipulation shares this idea of selling us a fake good, the end goal is the only thing that differs. Now that I have gone over the many ways that manipulators behave and act. I would like to dedicate the rest of this chapter on in-depth ways to defend yourself against each form of manipulation. With an understanding of the very basic ways to defend against manipulation, you are now equipped with the prerequisite knowledge required to hopefully avoid manipulation. As well as what to do when manipulation becomes unavoidable.

Let's start with emotional manipulation. We already understand that emotional manipulation is the act of someone trying to dictate and control how you feel. But how do you nip that behavior in the bud, so you can end or even perhaps avoid it? Allow me to use a hypothetical situation between two arguing lovers, as a training exercise in how to defuse a manipulator, as well as what behaviors within this scenario constitute emotional manipulation.

A man and his girlfriend have recently moved in with each other after dating for around three months. What drew this woman to this man is how he always seems to say the right thing, and always makes her feel good. Yet she cannot seem to shake the feeling that at times his platitudes are perhaps disingenuous. She also has begun to realize that her boyfriend is starting to slack off and not contribute to the rent of their shared apartment. She decides that she will sit down with him one day and discuss that perhaps it is time for him to get a job as to allow them to both maintain their current living arrangement. So the following day she sits down her boyfriend and says " Honey, I know you love me very much, but since we have moved in together I feel like you have somewhat been taking advantage of me, in the sense that you are not paying your share of rent here, and if we want to stay in this nice apartment than we both need to carry our weight."

Right as she completes her sentence her supposedly loving boyfriend begins to fly off the handle in what can best be described as rage, "Well your parents pay for everything, why should I be expected to get a job and pay when you have never worked for anything ever in your life. You know you're never going to find someone who loves you as much as me." Now before I dive further into this example allow me to provide some analysis of the behavior exhibited by the boyfriend, and why it is manipulative. In addition to how the girlfriend should appropriately respond to both de-escalate the situation and how she can avoid being manipulated further by him. To start first considering this, when most normal people are presented with an uncomfortable situation like this one where they perhaps could be in the wrong. Usually, their first reaction is to not fly into a rage. Most people will calmly listen to what is being presented to them and take it as such. In this case, we can see that the first thing the boyfriend did was get angry when presented with the possibility that he was in the wrong and as a result to try to deflect blame onto his girlfriend.

This projection took the form of him telling his girlfriend that he should not be asked to pay rent since she is already given money by her parents. This kind of behavior qualifies as manipulation because it sets up an unfair precedent for his convenience. He automatically assumes that since she is getting money for free then why should he be required to work and pay his fair share. The simple fact is that they both are in the apartment together and as a result both need to contribute equally if they want to stay together. By him getting irate at her and throwing abuse, he is trying to scare her into not pressing further with it, via the threat of ending the relationship.

For the girlfriend knowing how to react in this situation can seem to be very tricky, because on the one hand she loves her boyfriend and does not want him to leave her. On the other hand, thought him living rent-free in her apartment is just straight up unfair, so what should her course of action be? Well, the first step anyone should take when dealing with a manipulator, especially one who is prone to anger, is to keep their calm. If you can stay calm when presenting to a manipulator how their behavior is damaging than in a way you prevent further manipulation. From here the next step would be for her to make her boundaries very firm with her boyfriend. Saying something like this "If you are going to blow up at me when I try talking to you then there will be no relationship, and I am more than happy to just kick you out right now, with or without rent being paid."

The most important thing to remember when laying out firm boundaries is to follow up with them.

So, in this situation, she has laid out that if her boyfriend continues getting irate with her and being rude than she will just cut him off now. Here is where the problem lies, manipulators are excellent at getting someone to come back to them. In our example, it is very likely that even if she breaks it off with her boyfriend that he will come back and say to her. "Sorry honey I did not mean to blow up at you". Basically, telling her everything she wants to hear, and then when another incident between the two occurs he will promptly repeat the same behavior. That is why when dealing with a manipulator you must keep these boundaries firm and not falter or even give them an inch because they will take a mile. Now that we have gone over how to deal with manipulation in relationships. I would like to dive deeply into how the media uses manipulation to get us to purchase things, or even sway our opinion and how we can protect against it.

Take the mainstream news in the United States for example. Instead of reporting on simply just the news and happening events around the world. Certain news outlets will be composed of nothing but talking heads and editorials giving their opinion on everything. In a sense, they are trying to get you to think the way they want, whether this is out of malice or simple incompetence is up for debate. But the crux of the issue is that when a news story is reported today, it is no longer simply just "news" it is filled with many different people's opinions. And depending on the political leaning of the news outlet they may not report on other things. Another more damaging example of this kind of manipulation can be seen in social media such as Instagram and Facebook. And that is in the realm of the influencer, someone who is paid to present a false lifestyle and show off how certain products, whatever they may behave helped them attain it.

This form of manipulation preys on a common psychological trope and that is called the fear of missing out. When we see these people living super blessed lives and how they have everything one could want. We start feeling bad for ourselves and as a result, will go out and buy these products in the vain attempt that they will help us live the same kind of blessed life. The truth is that all sales try to get us to assume that our lives will be better with whatever product their pitching. Now that we know this how you can better equip yourself so that you do not fall victim to frivolous purchases of things you do not need. The first step in avoiding this type of manipulation is to take a glance back and realize, that what people post on social media is what they want you to see. In the same mindset that often what manipulators tell you is what they want you to hear. With that knowledge, you can better keep yourself from being swayed if you look at it like this. The second thing to understand is that if you do happen to decide to go and purchase the products, do research on them do not go and just buy something because it has Kylie Jenner's name stamped on it with a bunch of fabulous claims.

Always remember the truism that extraordinary claims require extraordinary facts. From there you can truly make an informed decision if you want to purchase something or not. If you have concluded that what someone is posting is a pure promotion or the product is harmful than drop that social media then and there, you're better off not following it, that will be your final solution if all else fails. Jumping back to media manipulation I would like to also talk about how advertisements try to use the same trick as social media influencers in getting us to purchase things that perhaps we do not need. I mentioned earlier in the book how whenever a new iPhone comes around apple the company that makes the iPhone will run a whole bunch of ads showing people from all walks of life in very happy scenarios with their fancy little iPhone. These ads are created this way to drive home the point that you can attain more happiness if you buy these items.

This feeds in on our desire to be like others and to also feed into our fear of missing out. This form of manipulation is also seen when we go to supermarkets with colorful ads and things that draw our attention from what matters. So, your best defense against these forms of manipulation is to research something before you buy it.

Too often than not we get convinced to buy something on emotional impulse and then try to justify it later. This is how we get manipulated we let our emotions override our logic and as a result, make incredibly poor decisions. To defend against this when shopping or trying to buy something always have an idea of what it is your buying and do not allow yourself to be swayed by mass advertising as if you do that you will be setting yourself up for a whole world of hurt and loss. Moving on from how salespeople try to manipulate you I would like to move back to emotional manipulation and how to defend against it. With some people, they will try to manipulate you within the confines of a romance while others such as friends or family. Will manipulate you within the confines of that already preexisting relationship. Simply put it can be easier for your friends and family to manipulate you because they do not have the issue of trying to get you in a relationship with them.

Manipulation in relationships are common places to spot them, yet the most unspoken relationship that manipulation persists is between family members. In most cases, relatives won't speak up against one another because since they're related by blood, they emotionally feel that it would be wrong to speak against them. Imagine this scenario; your cousin and his two children asked to move into your house, which you allow them to willingly. After some months go by, you notice that he has stopped paying rent, doesn't buy his groceries or utensils rather he uses your ingredients and your silverware.

You are being used.

So, you decide logically to bring up the fact that he is not carrying his weight in your house. So, you say "Hey cousin Tommy, I know you and your family have been hit by hard times, but if you are going to live within my home. Then you need to get a job and help contribute to bills and you know just carry your own". Keep in mind that when you brought this fact up to your cousin you said it very calmly and reasonably. If your cousin responds with "oh it's hard, working long hours at my job and school supplies for my kids. You understand right?" Your cousin's response indicates that your cousin has no incentive to pay any amount of money to you and they will continue leeching off you. By saying "you understand, right?" they are manipulating you to feel guilty for them and let them continue to abuse you and take advantage of you.

No – I what I understand is that you are not paying your expenses!

Make it clear that they will have to pay rent and if you want to compromise, they will be allowed to eat your food. If not, he will have to buy their own.

Conclusion

Throughout this book, we have discussed all of the things that are important to remember to avoid being manipulated, and to include positive persuasion in the way that you interact with others. It isn't something that is going to be achieved overnight, but with more and more practice, you can remember that you have what it takes to get the things that you desire most. The biggest mistake that some will make after learning of these methods is to use them to only their advantage and take from others rather than spreading the happiness and satisfaction received through influence. It is a lot easier to negatively manipulate someone than to positively persuade them. Sometimes, persuasion means building trust. Manipulation can simply mean instilling fear. While manipulation might be easier, it is going to cause a lot more difficult things in the end that you will have to clean up afterwards!

Remember that this process starts with really understanding someone's personality. There are common types of manipulators out there and you might be able to sense this personality trait in another person right away. Similarly, you will also recognize that there are hidden qualities that won't always emerge at first. Remember to recognize that not all manipulative behaviors presented by an individual indicates that she is a malicious person. Having manipulative parents or long-term partners can rub off on our behavior, so we might sometimes say and do things that aren't meant to be manipulative but can come off that way. Always look at intention when determining if someone is really being manipulative or not.

Also, don't forget that body language can play a huge role in how someone will be perceived. You can start to see persuasive body language in others more often than you did before as soon as you become aware of what this kind of body language looks like. Ensure you are aware of your own body language as well so as not to be manipulated by others.

At the end of the day, manipulation is generally a way for a person to get the things that they desire most. We all have basic human needs and instincts that drive our behavior. If we are not careful with how we go about getting these things, we can hurt others. The more equipped we are with the skills needed for positive influence, the easier it will be to achieve our deepest desires in a healthy way that benefits many.

To continue to grow your level of influence, remember that it starts with small moments of persuasion. Don't tell people what to do, encourage them from personal experience and stories learned from others. Don't try and trick someone into doing the things they don't want to do. Be honest with reward and consequence so that they can properly make the decision for themselves.

Always ensure that you are reflecting on your own behavior to make sure that you aren't going about things in the wrong way. With becoming influential, there is a certain level of confidence that comes along as well. If you are not careful, that confidence will drive you too far ahead of others, and you can get lost in what you perceive to be best for everyone. The better you can reflect and ensure you have the right intention, the easier it will be for others to be legitimately inspired by you. While it might be hard to do the right thing in times where what is easiest will also benefit you the most, remember to be empathetic towards others. Though it might be challenging, you will still ultimately get the things you desire most when you are doing so in a fair and rewarding way.

CPSIA information can be obtained
at www.ICGtesting.com
Printed in the USA
LVHW080721281220
674884LV00043B/417

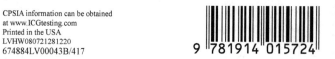